Language
and
Epilepsy

YVAN LEBRUN, PhD

Emeritus Professor of Neurolinguistics, Free University of Brussels, Belgium

and

FRANCO FABBRO, MD

Professor of Human Physiology, Research and Rehabilitation Centre Eugenio
Medea and University of Udine, Italy

W

WHURR PUBLISHERS
LONDON AND PHILADELPHIA

© 2002 Whurr Publishers

Whurr Publishers Ltd
19b Compton Terrace, London N1 2UN, England and
325 Chestnut Street, Philadelphia PA19106, USA

British Library Cataloguing in Publication Data

A catalogue record for this book is available from the
British Library.

ISBN 1 86156 312 4

Printed and bound in the UK by Athenaeum Press Limited,
Gateshead, Tyne & Wear.

Contents

Introduction

There are innumerable books on epilepsy. Many of them deal with the nature of the illness, its variegated symptomatology and/or its treatment. Others discuss the various subtypes of epilepsy and debate their classification. Still others describe the personal and social consequences of the illness.

Some of these numerous publications allude in passing to the verbal problems that epilepsy may entail. Others study in more detail the linguistic impairments observed in a particular subgroup of patients. But none, to the best of our knowledge, is entirely devoted to the many and complex relationships between epilepsy and verbal behaviour. The present monograph attempts to fill this gap by examining the various linguistic shortcomings, disorders, deviances and peculiarities that may be observed during or between seizures, and by trying to relate them to the disturbance of bioelectrical brain activity that is typical of epilepsy.

The terminology used in publications on epilepsy is far from being uniform, and so in the first chapter we have given a clear outline of the basic concepts of epileptology and have unequivocally defined the terms used to describe the various forms of epilepsy. The technique of electroencephalography employed to confirm diagnoses of epilepsy is summarized, and true epileptic seizures are contrasted with pseudo-seizures, i.e. accesses that clinically resemble genuine epileptic fits but do not correlate with paroxysmal discharges in the brain.

In Chapter 2, we show how the various names given to epilepsy in the past reflect the ideas, misconceptions and prejudices that were entertained about the illness. The names also tell of the saints who used to be invoked against epilepsy, and of the practices supposed to cure or avert it.

The third chapter, 'Ictal verbal behaviour', examines the various linguistic symptoms that patients may evidence during seizures, and shows how epileptic accesses at times interfere with patients' voluntary verbal behaviours and at other times elicit unintentional verbal utterances.

Chapter 4 examines which verbal behaviours are liable to trigger off epileptic attacks and under what circumstances. It also describes the symptoms of these reflex seizures and how the seizures can sometimes be avoided.

The relations between stuttering and epilepsy are still poorly understood, but we attempt to gain a better insight into these in Chapter 5.

Verbal impairments and deviations that can be observed in a number of patients between seizures and be reasonably related to their epilepsy are described in Chapter 6. This overview indicates that linguistic deficits concomitant with epilepsy are various and may be quite severe.

However, epilepsy is not incompatible with linguistic achievement, and this is discussed in Chapter 7. A number of people afflicted with epilepsy have produced literary masterpieces – and Saint Paul's epistles might not have been written if the apostle had not suffered from the falling sickness.

At times, epilepsy proves intractable, that is to say that all available antiepileptic drugs fail to reduce the number and/or severity of seizures. In such cases, neurosurgery is sometimes resorted to: part of the brain is removed or transected in an effort to alleviate the epilepsy and its negative consequences. Neurosurgery for the alleviation of intractable epilepsy is sometimes followed by transient or durable linguistic deficits and sometimes by an improvement of verbal behaviour. These changes are detailed in Chapter 8.

Because neurosurgery in the treatment of intractable epilepsy may have a durable negative influence on linguistic abilities, surgeons try to ascertain beforehand whether the cortical zone to be excised is essential for linguistic performance. To this end two different techniques may be used, hemispheric anaesthetization and cortical electrostimulation, which can only be used in conscious patients; Chapter 9 examines the verbal behaviour of patients as they are undergoing these two procedures.

Epilepsy may be accompanied by severe language disorders, particularly in children. Remediation of these disorders is dealt with in Chapter 10.

Finally, in Chapter 11, we draw some general conclusions following the investigation in the previous chapters of the many relationships between language and epilepsy.

Throughout the book a neurolinguistic methodology has been applied, which aims at an accurate description of linguistic phenomena due to cerebral damage or dysfunction. In this case, an effort has been made to detail the various verbal behaviours that can be observed in people suffering from epilepsy and which can reasonably be related to their illness. Unintentional and at times unconscious utterances have been distinguished from (impaired) deliberate performances. When appropriate, attention has been drawn to similar paroxysmal disorders occurring in neurological patients without epilepsy.

The various verbal manifestations are described and, where possible, an account is given of their likely pathogenesis. If different aetiopathological explanations have been proposed in the literature, they are discussed.

Due to its subject matter and its approach, this book addresses itself primarily to clinicians who are professionally concerned with epilepsy, such as neurologists, psychiatrists, paediatricians, neuropsychologists, and neurolinguists. However, it should also be of interest to general practitioners and to school physicians, as well as to parents and educators who have to care for children plagued with epilepsy. Hopefully, the book will help them better understand the linguistic difficulties these children are often confronted with and the strange verbal behaviours they sometimes exhibit, at times completely involuntarily. It will also alert them to the existence of subclinical epilepsy, which can be an unsuspected cause of specific language impairments or of learning disabilities.

With the lay readership in view, an effort has been made to use technical terms consistently and to clearly define or expound the anatomical and clinical notions used.

It is our hope that the book may contribute to a better understanding of epilepsy and thus help improve the lives of the many patients plagued with this illness.

Yvan Lebrun
Franco Fabbro

CHAPTER 1

The lexicon of epilepsy

Epilepsy is a cerebral disorder characterized by transitory but recurrent disturbances of the bio-electrical activity of the brain. The disturbance occurs in a number of neurones which suddenly start producing abnormal bursts. The pathological discharges may remain confined to these neurones or, on the contrary, spread to many other neurones, which in their turn start firing wildly. This wild firing is sometimes likened to a thunderstorm.

In a number of cases, the deviant electrical activity tends to originate each time at one particular place in the brain. This place is called an *epileptic* or *epileptogenic focus*. As long as the activity does not spread beyond the focus, the epilepsy is said to be *focal* or *local*. Focal epilepsies are often called after the cerebral lobe in which they take place, e.g. *temporal (lobe) epilepsy* or *frontal (lobe) epilepsy*. If the focus lies near the fissure of Rolando, the epilepsy is termed *Rolandic*.

In other cases, where many neurones located more or less symmetrically in the two cerebral hemispheres deliver pathological discharges simultaneously, the epilepsy is said to be *generalized*. At times, the abnormal bio-electrical activity is at first confined to a particular cerebral area and then, after a while, it starts spreading to other areas both in the same and in the contralateral hemisphere. This phenomenon is called *secondary generalization*. By contrast, generalized epilepsy not preceded by focal epilepsy is termed *primary generalized epilepsy*.

The Latin word *focus* means 'hearth', i.e. a fire confined within limits but with a potential danger of spreading more widely – an appropriate image of what may happen in epilepsy.

Symptomatic, idiopathic and cryptogenic epilepsy

The cause of the bio-electrical disorder may be an organic lesion or an inflammatory, circulatory, degenerative, metabolic or toxic affliction of the central nervous system. When this is the case, the epilepsy is said to be *symptomatic* or *secondary*.

In a number of patients, however, no local or general cause can be detected. If the patients do not evidence other neurological deficits, their epilepsy is considered *idiopathic*, i.e. due to some genetic or constitutional predisposition. In cases with idiopathic epilepsy, there is often a family history of similar ailments. Idiopathic epilepsy, which is also called *essential*, usually begins in childhood or adolescence, probably due to the fact that the maturing central nervous system is more prone than the fully mature brain to produce abnormal bio-electrical discharges.

At times, the causation of epilepsy cannot be discovered but accompanying deficits – for example, mental retardation – point to some cerebral damage. Epilepsy is then called *cryptogenic*, since its aetiology remains hidden. The response to medication in cryptogenic epilepsy tends to be less good than in idiopathic epilepsy.

Clinical versus subclinical epilepsy

In addition to pathological bio-electrical bursts in the brain, a number of patients present with transient abnormal motor behaviours or abnormal sensory or psychological experiences which result from the anomalous bio-electrical activity. These patients' epilepsy is called *clinical*. When epilepsy is not accompanied by abnormal motor, sensory or psychological phenomena, it is said to be *subclinical*.

Seizures

The abnormal movements, behaviours, sensations and moods associated with epileptic discharges are generically referred to as *seizures*, *attacks*, *fits*, *spells*, *accesses* or *episodes*. The words *ictus* and *paroxysm* may also be used. However, *paroxysm* sometimes denotes the climax of a seizure or an abnormal electrical discharge in the brain. And *ictus* is sometimes used to refer to a stroke, i.e. to a sudden cerebro-vascular accident such as a cerebral haemorrhage or a cerebral artery occlusion. Nonetheless, the adjectives derived from *ictus* are employed nearly exclusively in connection with epilepsy. *Ictal*, *pre-ictal*, *post-ictal*, and *inter-ictal* point to events occurring during, before, after or between seizures, respectively. *Paroxysmal* can be used as a synonym of *ictal*.

Status epilepticus

Seizures are normally of relatively short duration If this is not the case, i.e. if a seizure lasts unusually long, one speaks of *status epilepticus*. The Latin phrase is also used to refer to a fairly long series of seizures following rapidly upon one another with no return to normality between successive attacks. If recovery is achieved between fits occurring in sequence, one speaks of *serial epilepsy*.

Convulsive status epilepticus is a medical emergency, as it may lead to brain damage and even to death.

Ictal motor behaviour

A number of seizures are marked by abnormal motor events. Ictal motor behaviour may consist of a series of involuntary muscle contractions entailing fairly large movements: such contractions are called *convulsions*. Convulsions are generally bilateral, but may at times involve only one half of the body (*hemiconvulsions*). Convulsions taking place in the presence of high fever are named *febrile convulsions*; they are observed primarily in children.

Involuntary muscular contractions entailing movements of smaller amplitude are usually referred to as *myoclonias*. Movements of small amplitude occurring in only one body part are often designated as *jerks*. If only the fingers are affected, one speaks of *asterixis*.

In seizures of the *Jackson* (or *Bravais-Jackson*) *type* (also called *Jacksonian attacks*) the involuntary contractions occur in only one side of the body. They may be limited to a few muscles. If only one side of the face is involved, the seizure is termed *Rolandic*.

At times contractions begin in a limited area and then gradually spread to adjoining areas so as to finally involve a whole limb or a whole body half. Such a spread is called *Jacksonian march*. When a Jacksonian seizure lasts unusually long, it is sometimes referred to as *epilepsia partialis continua*.

If muscular contractions are bilateral and more or less symmetrical, the seizure is designated as *myoclonic*.

After a motor episode, there may be transient paralysis of the muscles that were involuntarily contracted. This palsy is called *Todd's paralysis*.

There are epileptic attacks during which the head or the eyes or both are deviated to one side. If it is the side where the epileptic focus is located in the brain, the seizure is called *ipsiversive*, and patients are said to be looking at their focus. If the head or the eyes turn to the opposite side, the seizure is regarded as *adversive* or *contraversive*. At times, the whole body is turned to one side; patients start whirling until they fall to the ground. Such seizures are called *gyratory*.

Some motor seizures are marked by a sustained contraction of the musculature. Usually there is rigid extension of all four limbs and there may be *opisthotonos*, i.e. an arched position of the body, which rests on the head and heels. Such seizures are *tonic*. *Clonic* seizures, on the contrary, are characterized by repetitive muscle contractions. In young children, these contractions are often termed *infantile spasms*. They are typical of a form of epilepsy named *West's syndrome*, after Dr West who described this form of epilepsy in his own child in 1841. When infantile spasms affect head, arm and trunk muscles, they may cause repeated flexions which somewhat resemble Eastern salutations and are therefore called *salaam attacks*.

In children with the *Lennox-Gastaut syndrome* (after two well-known epileptologists, William Lennox and Henri Gastaut), seizures are often characterized by a stare, a jerk and/or a fall: the child has a fixed gaze, performs an involuntary movement and/or loses his/her balance. Occasionally, tonic spasms are observed, more likely during sleep. A number of children with West's syndrome progress to the Lennox-Gastaut syndrome. The syndrome is considered a *malignant* form of childhood epilepsy, because it is often therapy-resistant and is frequently accompanied by mental retardation. By contrast, forms of childhood epilepsy that tend to pass spontaneously or can be medically controlled and are not concomitant with intellectual deficiency are said to be *benign*.

Tonico-clonic seizures combine tonic and clonic features. They are typical of *grand mal* episodes. In grand mal seizures patients lose consciousness and fall to the ground. They may let out a yell, the so-called *initial epileptic cry*. There ensues a generalized tonic contraction of the musculature with apnoea, i.e. arrest of respiration. The upper limbs are generally flexed while the lower limbs are extended. After a short while, the sustained muscular contraction gives way to a quick succession of contractions and relaxations causing clonic movements. During the clonic phase, the tongue may be bitten, and foaming at the mouth may occur. The foam may contain blood if patients have bitten themselves. Also, in many cases urine is passed. Respiration is re-established but may be stertorous, i.e. accompanied by a harsh snoring or rasping sound. Towards the end of the clonic phase, the intervals between the muscular contractions become longer, and the involuntary movements finally abate. Patients remain unconscious for a variable period of time. On recovering awareness, they may feel tired or stiff all over. There may be temporary dizziness. Not infrequently, patients sleep for several hours after the attack. Grand mal seizures are regarded as *major* epileptic fits.

Atonic seizures are characterized by a loss of postural tonus, which may cause sudden dropping of the head or a sudden fall. In the latter case, the seizure is occasionally called a *drop attack*. If the patient remains immobile on the floor for a while, the attack may be said to be *akinetic*.

During seizures, iterative movements mimicking simple actions such as chewing, scratching, rubbing, fidgeting or walking are sometimes observed. These movements are called *automatisms*. Occasionally, the automatic action consists of laughing or crying. Bouts of ictal laughing are referred to as *gelastic*, while bouts of ictal crying are named *dacrystic* or *quiritarian*.

If some seemingly purposeful action is involuntarily performed, the seizure is said to be *psychomotor*. The ictal activity may vary from fit to fit or be stereotyped, i.e. repeat itself from one attack to the next. When violent or aggressive behaviour is observed during a seizure, the patient is considered to have *raptus epilepticus*. It may also happen that during psychomotor seizures the patients continue the actions they were engaged in when the seizures started. However, the ictal performance is likely to be erratic or deviant. Psychomotor seizures may be accompanied by involuntary repetitive muscle contractions (*focal cloni*) or by head turning or eye deviation.

Because psychomotor seizures occur primarily in temporal lobe epilepsy, some clinicians use the phrase *psychomotor epilepsy* to refer to temporal (lobe) epilepsy.

Ictal sensory or psychic experiences

During seizures, patients may feel all sorts of sensations and experience various kinds of moods. The ictal sensations may be illusionary. Patients may seem to be seeing brilliant spots (*phosphenes*) or to be hearing sounds (*acousmas*). They may also have *paresthesias*, i.e. bodily sensations without actual stimuli. Sensations may also be distorted. Objects looked at may appear unusually small (*micropsia*), inordinately large (*macropsia*) or misshapen (*metamorphopsia*). The visual sensations may continue after the objects have been removed from sight (*palinopsia*).

There may also be somato-sensory experiences. Patients may feel epigastric or abdominal pain or have an impression of constriction (somewhere) in their body.

Patients may also have hallucinations, which may be uni- or multi-sensorial. They may see scenes that appear quite familiar, as if they had witnessed them before (an impression of *déjà-vu*). Conversely, the scenes may look completely strange and give rise to an impression of *jamais-vu*.

Hallucination may also concern the patient's own body, which may feel amputated or shorter or larger than it is in reality.

Hallucinatory experiences may be stereotyped or vary from one spell to the next. Patients may or may not be aware that they are having hallucinations, i.e. they may not realize that what they are perceiving does not correspond to external reality.

If patients experience strange moods or go through trance-like or dreamy states or have a sense of unreality, depersonalization or disembodiment, the seizure is called *psychic*. During psychic seizures patients not infrequently feel fearful or even terrified. At times, however, they feel ecstatically happy.

Hallucinations and psychic states not accompanied by symptoms that an observer can perceive, are often called *équivalents épileptiques* or *équivalents comitiaux* (ictal equivalents) by French neurologists. Formerly, the phrases *épilepsie larvée* (masked epilepsy) and *épilepsie non-convulsivante* (non-convulsive epilepsy) were used.

Consciousness

There are seizures during which consciousness is preserved: patients remain aware of their environment and realize that they are having an attack. Such seizures are called *simple partial*, and after a simple partial fit, patients can usually remember all that happened during the fit.

There are also seizures during which consciousness is impaired: patients are unresponsive to stimulation, and post-ictally they are amnesic about what happened during the episode. Such seizures with alteration of consciousness are called *complex partial*. A simple partial attack may evolve into a complex partial attack, i.e. awareness may at first be preserved and then become impaired.

Occasionally, contact with the environment is preserved during the seizure, and yet afterwards patients prove amnesic for (most of) what happened while they were having the attack. Contact with the environment is usually considered to be maintained if patients answer questions or follow verbal instructions. It is retrospectively considered to have been preserved in patients who, though they failed during the seizure to react to verbal stimulation, are able afterwards to remember the questions they were asked or the instructions they were given.

Absences are sudden and short-lived spells with clouding of consciousness. Patients generally fail to react to stimulation. They interrupt the activity they were involved in when the seizure started, or they proceed with it in a sluggish or inappropriate way. They may stare into space or blink repeatedly or perform automatisms. Following the absence there is rapid recovery of consciousness. Patients usually resume the interrupted activity. They may not be aware of having gone through a blank spell.

Absences are often referred to as *petit mal epilepsy*. In children they may occur a great many times a day. They are then named *pyknolepsy* (from the Greek *pykno-*, dense).

In grand mal seizures consciousness is completely lost. Other motor seizures may also at times be accompanied by total loss of awareness.

Aura

Before they lose consciousness or become unresponsive, patients may experience sensations or moods (such as fear) which remain fairly constant from seizure to seizure and which they may therefore learn to recognize as the initial symptoms of a fit. These symptoms form the *aura*. The word *aura* originally meant 'air, wind, zephyr'. It was applied to the introductory ictal symptoms by the Greek physician Galen after he had heard an epileptic boy liken the sensation which he would feel just before losing consciousness to a cold breeze blowing upon a part of his body.

During the aura patients may involuntarily start running, and continue to run until they fall unconscious. This behaviour is called *cursive epilepsy*. The phrase may also be used when running is observed during a psychomotor fit.

Some epileptologists apply the word *aura* also to somato-sensory and to psychic seizures, probably because it is not always easy to distinguish an aura ushering in a primary generalized seizure from a sensory or psychic attack immediately followed by a secondary generalization with loss of consciousness. A second reason is that occasionally a seizure ceases after the aura: the introductory sensory or psychic symptoms are not followed by others, and thus the access is abortive.

Patients experiencing an aura (in its narrow sense) may tell a person they are about to have a seizure. If a psychomotor or generalized convulsive attack actually takes place and is rather severe, patients may afterwards prove amnesic for the aura and the statement made during it, that is, they may not remember having experienced introductory symptoms and having told someone about it.

Reflex epilepsy

Some epileptic accesses are regularly triggered off by a specific and identifiable stimulus. As the triggering stimulus is often a sensation and as the epileptic response may be motor, the whole mechanism has been viewed as a sort of reflex and the corresponding type of epilepsy been termed *reflex epilepsy*.

Actually, in reflex epilepsy, the precipitant may be a sensation more or less passively experienced by the patients (such as hearing a particular type of noise) or an action performed by them (such as solving mathematical problems). As an example of reflex epilepsy triggered off by a specific type of visual sensation *television epilepsy* may be quoted. Seizures brought on by the flickering TV light are generally of the tonic-clonic type.

In a number of patients, myoclonic or atonic seizures are provoked by sudden auditory or visual stimuli, such as unexpected bangs or flashes of light likely to produce a startle reaction in the healthy. This type of reflex epilepsy is therefore termed *startle epilepsy*.

Prodromal symptoms

During the hours or even the days that immediately precede an epileptic seizure, patients may exhibit abnormal movements, peculiar moods or unusual behaviours. The patients or their relatives may come to recognize these prodromal signs and thus sense when a seizure is building up.

Table 1.1 Synopsis of the most frequent types of epilepsy and seizures

A 1. *Generalized epilepsy*
       Many neurones in the two cerebral hemispheres fire abnormal discharges
       simultaneously
   2. *Focal* (or *local*) *epilepsy*
       Epileptic discharges remain confined to a limited cerebral area

B 1. *Symptomatic* (or *secondary*) *epilepsy*
       Due to some detectable structural, infectious or metabolic
       derangement of the central nervous system
   2. *Idiopathic* (or *constitutional* or *essential*) *epilepsy*
       No lesion or affection can be discovered that could legitimately be held
       responsible for the epilepsy
   3. *Cryptogenic epilepsy*
       No direct cause can be detected but there is evidence of cerebral damage

C 1. *Subclinical epilepsy*
       Pathological bio-electrical discharges in the brain without abnormal motor
       behaviour or abnormal sensory or psychic experiences
   2. *Clinical epilepsy*
       Transient abnormal motor behaviours or abnormal sensory or psychic experiences
       in addition to pathological bio-electrical discharges in the brain

D 1. *Motor seizures*
       Grand mal seizures
       Myoclonic seizures
       Bravais-Jackson seizures
       Versive seizures
       Gyratory seizures
       Tonic seizures
       Clonic seizures
       Atonic and akinetic seizures
       Psychomotor seizures
   2. *(Somato-)sensory seizures*
   3. *Psychic seizures*

E 1. *Simple partial seizures*
       Consciousness is preserved
   2. *Complex partial seizures*
       Consciousness is impaired
   3. *Grand mal seizures and a number of other motor seizures*
       Consciousness is lost

F   *Generalized seizures*
       Grand mal seizures
       Myoclonic seizures

(contd)

Table 1.1 (contd)

Tonic and clonic seizures
Atonic seizures
Absences

Note: many patients with epilepsy experience more than just one type of seizure. Moreover, partial seizures not infrequently evolve into secondary generalized attacks.

Electroencephalography

The bio-electrical anomalies typical of epilepsy can be recorded by means of electrodes placed on the scalp or, in exceptional cases, laid directly on the cortex (subdural electrodes) or implanted in the brain tissue (depth electrodes). A surgical procedure is required to position electrodes on the cerebral cortex or in cerebral structures. Subdural electrodes are usually several in number, forming a strip or a grid or sheet. The strips can usually be introduced through burr holes. The placement of larger sheets necessitates a craniotomy. Depth electrodes are thin multicontact shafts.

The technique by means of which the bio-electrical activity of the brain can be recorded is called *electroencephalography*. If the electrodes are on the scalp, one speaks of *surface electroencephalography*. If they lie on the cortex, the recording technique is called *electrocorticography*. If the electrodes are implanted in the brain, one speaks of *stereo-electroencephalography*.

Usually, the electrodes are connected by wires to the registering device. In *telemetric* electroencephalography, however, the wires are replaced by radio transmission, so that the patient can move about while the bio-electrical activity is being recorded.

If patients are filmed during the recording of their bio-electrical brain activity, one speaks of *video-electroencephalography*. This technique is particularly useful if one wants to correlate the patients' clinical manifestations with the abnormal brain activity.

In electroencephalographic recordings, which are called *encephalograms* or *EEGs*, epileptic discharges usually show as spikes or as slow waves or as a combination of both (so-called *spike-wave complexes*). These anomalies may be isolated, irregular, or synchronous (occurring simultaneously at various places in the brain).

If the EEG is recorded during a seizure, it usually shows bio-electrical abnormalities. In seizures with involuntary muscle contractions, the electrical bursts recorded in the EEG are often synchronous with the contractions.

In generalized seizures, numerous simultaneous discharges are recorded over the two cerebral hemispheres. If they are present from the beginning of the seizure, they are said to be *ambincipient*, i.e. starting at the same time on both sides of the brain. EEGs made during grand mal seizures, during myoclonic, tonic or atonic seizures and also during absences show the typical ambincipient pattern of primary generalized seizures.

Inter-ictally, when patients with epilepsy rest quietly without being asleep, the EEG may show sporadic pathological discharges or, on the contrary, look normal. When a person is suspect of epilepsy and their rest EEG does not evidence anomalous electrical activity, one often resorts to (drug-induced) sleep, hyperventilation (overbreathing) or intermittent photic stimulation. These provocative manoeuvres are known to elicit abnormal electrical signs in subjects having epilepsy. In this way, the physician's suspicion that the patient may suffer from epilepsy can often be confirmed.

The EEG of children with West's syndrome usually shows a pattern of almost continuous and irregular slow spikes and waves which has been given the name of *hypsarrhythmia*.

In some other children, sustained abnormal bio-electrical brain activity can be recorded during certain phases of sleep. This anomaly used to be called *(electrical) status epilepticus during sleep*. The current name is *syndrome of continuous spikes and waves during (slow) sleep*, often abbreviated as CSWS. The nocturnal discharges may remain confined to a particular cerebral area or, on the contrary, show in most of the brain.

In a number of patients, epileptiform discharges unaccompanied by clinical manifestations occur in the waking state. Some of these patients have clinical seizures in addition and are therefore known to suffer from epilepsy. Others, on the contrary, never have clinical seizures. As a consequence, their subclinical epilepsy may not be discovered until an EEG examination is finally performed.

Non-epileptic paroxysms

For diagnostic and therapeutic purposes epileptic seizures need to be distinguished from paroxysmal occurrences which clinically resemble epileptic seizures but do not correlate with epileptic brain activity.

Psychic trauma and emotional stress may entail motor seizures during which patients fall to the floor (generally without hurting themselves), flail their arms and legs in an incoordinate way, arch their back while resting on heels and occiput (so-called *opisthotonos*), roll from side to side, show pelvic thrusting, shout, cry, gasp or retch. They may seem unconscious. However, they may strike out or bite if one attempts to restrain them. On recovering from this state of agitation, they generally claim to have no recollection of it.

Such convulsive accesses somewhat resemble grand mal or myoclonic attacks. They are sometimes called *hysterical*. They occur more frequently in women than in men. In earlier times they were thought to affect only females and to be due to wanderings of the womb (in Greek *hustera*) in the body. Actually, in women these fits not infrequently appear to originate from rape or sexual abuse. If they are prolonged, they may be mistaken for status epilepticus.

At times, bouts of collective convulsive hysteria are observed. For example, episodes of severe agitation resembling convulsions were noted in a number of French Jansenists in the first part of the eighteenth century. Attacks usually occurred when the believers visited the tomb of their coreligionist François de Pâris (1690–1727) in the Saint-Médard cemetery, which for that reason the Archbishop of Paris ordered to be closed (1732). The Jansenists presenting with such fits were called *convulsionnaires*.

On the other hand, anxiety may cause swoons. Patients collapse, usually without injury, and lie apparently unconscious for varying periods of time. There are no convulsive movements. The musculature is often flaccid. Such seizures are reminiscent of atonic or akinetic attacks. They too occur more frequently in women.

Panic attacks, possibly with a sense of depersonalization or unreality sometimes occur in individuals with phobias as well as in patients with disturbances of the cardiac rhythm. Such attacks may be mistaken for psychic epileptic seizures.

Anger or frustration may result in tantrums during which patients shout, thrash about and evidence aggressive or destructive behaviour. These tantrums may masquerade as raptus epilepticus. They tend to occur primarily in patients with personality disorders or mental retardation.

These various sorts of psychogenic attacks are generically referred to as *pseudo-seizures*.

Distinguishing between pseudo-seizures and truly epileptic seizures may be difficult, as there are patients who present with both types of paroxysms: they suffer from epilepsy as well as from a psychiatric disorder causing pseudo-seizures. There are also patients whose epileptic attacks are not infrequently induced by stressful situations or by strong or unpleasant affects, thus falsely giving the impression that they are psychogenic in nature.

Epileptic seizures need to be distinguished not only from pseudo-seizures but also from paroxysmal episodes caused by a number of neurological affections. As a matter of fact, some disorders of the central nervous system entail sudden falls resembling epileptic motor fits. For instance, transient ischemic accidents (TIA), which are short-lived perturbations of the blood circulation in the brain, may cause patients to fall to the floor (so-called *drop attacks*).

Hyperekplexia or startle disorder may entail falls resembling those of startle epilepsy. Hyperekplectic patients are unusually sensitive to sudden sensory stimulation: unexpected noises, flashes of light or bodily contacts elicit in them an intense startle, possibly resulting in a fall.

Reduction in blood supply to the brain may cause syncope. The loss of consciousness may resemble that of generalized seizures. And if the reduction in blood supply is prolonged, convulsions may occur.

Food poisoning such as *ergotism*, which results from eating rye bread infected with a fungus called *ergot*, may also bring on convulsions (see p. 23).

There are also non-pathological manifestations which may be mistaken for epileptic attacks. For instance, involuntary muscle contractions and motor tics (unintentional, repetitive, stereotyped, aimless movements) are observed in many healthy children. Brief episodes of shuddering or shivering with stiffness or tremor may occur too. They are benign and generally disappear spontaneously as the child grows older.

Daydreaming is common, particularly in bored children, and should not be confused with epileptic absences.

Finally, mention may be made of individuals simulating epilepsy. They malinger because they seek financial compensation (for instance, after an accident), try to gain sympathy or attention, or want to escape environmental challenges or demands. Before the advent of electroencephalography, conscripts sometimes feigned epilepsy to be exempted from military service.

Epilepsy, then, needs to be distinguished from a variety of psychiatric or neurological disorders as well as from a number of non-pathological behaviours. Differential diagnosis rests on EEG recordings, careful clinical examination and detailed history taking.

Treatment

Epilepsy is usually treated by means of antiepileptic drugs generically called *anticonvulsants*. The major anticonvulsants are phenobarbital (introduced by Hauptmann in 1912 to replace bromides which were extensively used in the nineteenth century), phenytoin or diphenylhydantoin (introduced by Putnam and Merritt in 1937), pheneturide, carbamazepine (introduced in 1960), sodium valproate (introduced in 1963) and valproic acid, ethosuximide, primidone (a barbiturate like phenobarbital), progabide, vigabatrin, and lamotrigin, as well as a number of benzodiazepines such as clobazam, clonazepam, and diazepam. At times, the drugs are administered singly (monotherapy). In other cases, a few of them are combined (polytherapy).

CHAPTER 2

The names of epilepsy

Introduction

In one of his shorter dialogues, the Greek philosopher Plato dealt with the question of whether names are significant by nature or by convention. Is there some specific appropriateness of the sounds of names to the named objects or are names arbitrary designations? Plato seems to have favoured the former view. Nowadays, however, there is general agreement that there is no necessary bond between a word and the thing named by this word.

Yet the word may reflect some aspects of the thing. In particular, it may be reminiscent of the beliefs and prejudices that were, or still are, entertained about the thing. The vocabulary is often the repository of old persuasions and obsolete views. It bears the mark of ancient opinions and bygone theories. It carries vestigial patterns of thought once dominant. Thus, the popular names of diseases often reflect the awe the diseases used to inspire and the views that were held regarding their nature and origin. Epilepsy is a striking example of this. The various appellations of the illness remind one of the many ideas and superstitions it has given rise to. Indeed, there are few other ailments whose names speak so clearly about past conceptions and misconceptions.

Sacred disease

From time immemorial epilepsy has been considered a special disease, a weird illness, a strange malady. The ancients thought that it was inflicted on humans by the gods. Hence the title *The Sacred Disease* which Hippocrates gave to the book in which he dealt with epilepsy. Yet the Greek physician did not himself think that epileptic seizures had a divine origin. In the introduction to his book he wrote:

> I am about to discuss the disease called 'sacred'. It is not, in my opinion, any more
> divine or more sacred than other diseases, but has a natural cause, and its

13

supposed divine origin is due to men's inexperience, and to their wonder at its peculiar character.

As a matter of fact, Hippocrates and his school thought epilepsy to be due to an excess of phlegm (one of the four body humours) overflowing the brain.

The Hippocratic view of epilepsy was not accepted, and for centuries the disease continued to be regarded as a sickness of supernatural origin. The Romans called it *morbus sacer, morbus divinus* or *lues deifica*, i.e. the sacred disease or the divine plague. In French it was referred to as *mal sacré, mal sainct, mal divin* or *haut mal*. The Germans spoke of *heilige Krankheit, heiliges Web* – sacred disease – or *das Höchste* – the supreme. In the dialect of Mecklenburg, the disease used to be called *dat billig* – the holy (disease).

In ancient Rome, if someone had a seizure during a *comitia*, i.e. an assembly of the people, the assembly had to be dispersed, because the occurrence of the seizure was considered an ominous sign. Epilepsy, therefore, was often called *morbus comitialis*. The adjective *comitial* is still used in French medical jargon when discussing epilepsy. In Italian, the Roman appellation survives as *morbo comiziale*.

The supernatural origin of epilepsy was at times regarded as diabolic. Not infrequently people suffering from epilepsy were considered to be possessed of a demon. In Greek, *epileptos* meant not only 'epileptic' but also 'controlled by an evil spirit'. The Gospels relate that Jesus cured an epileptic boy by exorcising him, i.e. by forcing the devil to leave the boy's body. This is how Luke (9: 37–42) tells the story, which is also found in Matthew (17: 14–18) and in Mark (9: 17–27):

> And it came to pass, that on the next day, when they were come down from the hill, much people met him. And, behold, a man of the company cried out, saying, Master, I beseech thee, look upon my son: for he is mine only child. And, lo, a spirit taketh him, and he suddenly crieth out; and it teareth him that he foameth again, and bruising him hardly departeth from him . . . And Jesus answering said, . . . Bring thy son hither. And as he was yet a coming, the devil threw him down, and tare him. And Jesus rebuked the unclean spirit, and healed the child, and delivered him again to his father.

Several saints, including St Germain, the fifth-century bishop of Auxerre, France, and St Ignatius de Loyola, the sixteenth-century founder of the Jesuits, are reported to have imitated Jesus and to have cured persons with epilepsy by driving out the devil tormenting them.

In old Egypt, patients were advised to eat donkey excrement diluted in wine. The purpose was to sicken the demon inside and cause him to leave the sufferer's body. In some places in India they would apply a red-hot iron to the forehead of patients to chase off the evil spirit. In Europe, a hole was sometimes bored in the skull to let out the devil.

Because people afflicted with epilepsy were often considered to be possessed, epilepsy was called *le mauvais mal* or *la male passion* (the wicked disease) in French, and *böses Wesen* (wicked spirit) in German.

The demons or fiends causing epilepsy were generally assumed to be deaf and dumb on account of the fact that during seizures patients often fail to react to verbal stimuli and do not speak.

However, at times, patients were submitted to cauterization or trepanation not to rid them of a demon but rather to restore a humoral balance in the head. Ancient and medieval medicine believed that the human body contained four fluids: blood, bile, black choler and phlegm. These cardinal humours had to be present in well-defined proportions, and an excess of any of them could result in disease. Epilepsy was caused by an excessive quantity of phlegm – supposed to be the coldest of the four fluids – or of phlegm mixed with air, in the brain. Cauterization, i.e. application of a hot iron on some part of the head, was aimed at counteracting the coldness of the offending humour, whereas trepanation was expected to provide an outlet for the excessive mixture of air and phlegm.

Lunar disease

Epilepsy was also ascribed to the pernicious influence of the moon. It was therefore called *morbus lunaticus* or *morbus astralis* in Latin, *mal lunatique* in French, and *maanziekte* (moon sickness) in Dutch. In Greek, *seleniakos* – an adjective derived from *selene* (moon) – meant 'epileptic'. The chapters in the Gospel by St Luke and by St Matthew which recount the healing of an epileptic boy by Jesus are entitled in the King James version *He heals a* (or *the*) *lunatick*. In Anglo-Saxon countries, people with epilepsy were often said to be *moonstruck*.

In the nineteenth century, a beverage supposed to be efficacious against epilepsy was given twice a year to sufferers in Tain-L'Hermitage on the river Rhone in France. The drug, which was called *le grand remède* (the great remedy), had to be taken when the moon was full. The *grand remède* used to be prepared with white cheese-rennet. Nowadays, a potion is still sold in and around Tain-L'Hermitage under the name of *Grand Remède de l'Hermitage*, but it contains more bromide than cheese-rennet. Bromides are the first drugs to have been used with some success against epilepsy, but they had adverse side-effects.

The association of epilepsy with the moon and more specifically with lunar cycles (which are about four weeks in duration) may be due in part to the fact that in a number of females suffering from epilepsy attacks occur only, or increase in frequency, during menstrual periods. In this connection it may be recalled that the word *menses*, which means 'menstruation', originally meant 'months' and is akin to Greek *men* (month) and *mene* (moon).

Infamous disease

Persons with epilepsy were often debarred from a number of positions or privileges. Not until the reformation of the canon law in 1983 could a man afflicted with epilepsy be ordained as a priest. In early Christian times, patients were refused holy communion. In many places the sale of a slave was void if the slave turned out to suffer from epilepsy.

Because the disease was so infamous, some of the sufferers who came to Tain-L'Hermitage to drink the great remedy wore masks in order to conceal their identities.

Contagious disease

Epilepsy was often considered contagious. People therefore used to spit on patients to protect themselves from the illness, and for this reason another name for the disease was *morbus insputatus* (the disease you spit at) in Latin. The Romans used to plant a nail where a person with epilepsy had fallen in order to prevent the disease from propagating. The idea was to pin to the spot the evil spirit causing the convulsions.

In the second half of the nineteenth century, the inhabitants of Tain-L'Hermitage campaigned for the closing down of the hospital for people with epilepsy run by the Count of Larnage in their town. They were afraid of being contaminated by the inmates of the hospital.

Patients with epilepsy used to be confined with the insane. Esquirol, a nineteenth century physician, pleaded for the establishment of special divisions for epileptics. However, he was motivated by solicitude for the insane rather than by a concern for those afflicted with epilepsy. He believed, as many had done before him, that the mere sight of an epileptic attack might render a healthy person epileptic. Since the mentally deranged, he thought, were more impressionable than healthy people, the likelihood of their becoming epileptic after witnessing a seizure was even greater. Accordingly, he recommended that people with epilepsy should be confined separately to minimize the danger to other patients.

This misconception – that looking at an ill person is often enough to catch their disease – is actually a very old one, and arises from the notion that the gaze establishes a contact: by setting eyes on someone, you get in touch with them. However, people said that patients with epilepsy could also infect others with their breath or with their sweat. Therefore, it was dangerous not only to look at sufferers having a convulsive seizure but also to approach them or touch them.

Hereditary disease

Epilepsy was also held to be hereditary. This is why, in various countries, people plagued by epilepsy were not allowed to marry. In some parts of India, a marriage can still be made void if it appears that one of the partners had epilepsy before getting married, but concealed the fact.

Delinquency

Sufferers from epilepsy were suspected of all sorts of misdeeds. Up until the end of the nineteenth century, sexual deviance, pyromania and criminalism were frequently thought to be associated with epilepsy.

Geniality and religiosity

However, at times epilepsy was regarded as a sign of special endowment. Patients were occasionally considered to be soothsayers or prophets. They were thought to have visions and to be able to foresee future events.

Paroxysmal attacks were sometimes deemed to be of the same nature as moments of artistic inspiration. Indeed, based on the Latin adage *nullum ingenium magnum sine mixtura dementiae* (there can be no great genius without some degree of insanity) the view was now and then put forward that artistic talent was due to epilepsy.

People with epilepsy were also held to be prone to religious conversion. St Paul's sudden persuasion to Christianity on the way to Damascus has sometimes been ascribed to epilepsy.

Hyper-religiosity is still considered by a number of experts to be a personality trait of patients with temporal epilepsy. The religious concerns of Mohammed, the founder of Islam, and of Vincent Van Gogh, the now much celebrated nineteenth-century painter who was for a time a zealous evangelist, are thought by some to be due, at least in part, to epilepsy. Foote-Smith and Bayne (1991) have submitted that the disease may also have been responsible for Joan of Arc's visions as well as for her strong religious conviction.

Dreadful disease

Epilepsy was dreaded. Therefore its name was taboo in many quarters. Euphemisms had to be used instead, and often had a propitiatory function. For instance, the French spoke of the *beau mal* (the nice disease) or *bon mal* (the good disease). At times, they simply referred to the illness as *le mal* (the disease).

Epilepsy was – and still is – a serious handicap, hence its Latin names *morbus sonticus* (severe illness) and *morbus maior* (great disease). The French spoke of *grande maladie*, *grand mal* or *gros mal* (fateful disease), and the Germans of *schwere Not* (great predicament). *Grand mal* is still used to denote a major form of epilepsy (see p. 4).

Falling sickness

Sudden falls were considered the hallmark of epilepsy. Accordingly, the disease was often called *falling sickness*, *falling ill* or *falling evil*. The Romans used *morbus caducus* and *passio caduca*, the French *mal caduc*, the Italians *mal caduco*, the Dutch *vallende ziekte*, *vallend euvel*, *vallende krankte* or *vallende zucht*, and the Germans *die Fallsucht*, *die fallende Sucht*, *das fallende Leid*, *die fallende Krankheit*, or simply *das Fallende*. In old French, the condition was defined as *le mal de quoi l'on chiet* (the disease that causes you to fall). In Gaelic it is called *galar titimeach*, i.e. 'the falling disease'. In Walloon dialects, *toumer di grand mâ* (to fall due to grand mal) is the same as 'to have a convulsive seizure'.

In French, epilepsy was also named *mal de terre*, i.e. 'ground or earth disease', maybe because sufferers fall to the ground.

Cramps

Convulsions are a striking feature of some forms of epilepsy. Therefore the word *cramp* was sometimes used to denote the condition. A *cramp-ring* was a ring assumed to be efficacious against cramps, i.e. epilepsy, especially if it had been hallowed by the king on Good Friday. In fact, the king of England was sometimes considered able to cure epilepsy, much as the king of France was thought to be able to heal scrofula (which for that reason was often termed *king's evil*).

In slang, epilepsy was sometimes called *crank*. A *counterfeit crank* was a rogue who feigned epilepsy in order to move compassion or get money. The sixteenth century French physician Ambroise Paré refers to these swindlers, indicating that some of them put soap in their mouths to imitate the foam that may come from the lips of sufferers when they have a grand mal attack.

Epilepsy

As for the word *epilepsy* itself, it derives from Latin *epilepsia*, which is akin to the Greek verb *epilambanein*, 'to take hold of, to seize'. The image survives in the English word *seizure*, which denotes an attack of epilepsy. The word *epilepsy* was introduced into the English vocabulary in the sixteenth century, and replaced the former *epilency*.

For a long time, *epilepsy* and its popular synonyms were used to refer nearly exclusively to motor seizures, particularly grand mal convulsions. The epileptic nature of sensory or psychic attacks was not recognized, and the strange behaviour of patients during psychomotor accesses was most of the time ascribed to madness. On the other hand, the tonic and clonic muscle contractions caused by epilepsy could not be clearly distinguished from other types of involuntary muscular contractions or from cramps.

Epilepsy and hysteria

Before the advent of electroencephalography it was at times difficult to discriminate between epilepsy and hysteria. Moreover, it was believed that some patients suffered from both epilepsy and hysteria, and that the two diseases could concur to bring on complex seizures. It was also assumed that hysteria could easily evolve into epilepsy causing *epilepsia uterina* or *epilepsia hysterica*.

Convulsive hysteria can be contagious. Instances of hysterical epidemics have been recorded, e.g. the convulsionists of the Saint-Médard cemetery (see p. 11). Such outbreaks were sometimes called *imitative hysteria* because it was realized that conscious or unconscious imitation played an important part in their occurrence. Another name was *chorea imitativa*, due to the confusion between epilepsy, hysteria and chorea.

Hercules and St Paul

A number of celebrities were, or are supposed to have been, afflicted with epilepsy. The list includes the Greek demi-god Hercules. According to Greek mythology, Hercules killed his music teacher Linos and later slaughtered his own wife and children during what may have been episodes of raptus epilepticus (see above pp. 4–5). In Latin, *morbus herculeus* or *herculanus*, i.e. Hercules' disease or Herculean disease, was one of the many names given to epilepsy. Hercules was sometimes called *Alcides* and thus in French both *mal herculéen* and *mal d'Alcide* are occasionally used to refer to epilepsy.

St Paul too is thought to have suffered from epilepsy. In Gaelic, the illness is therefore sometimes called *galar Phoel*, i.e. 'Paul's disease'.

Saints against the disease

Because epilepsy is a severe condition and for centuries there existed no really efficient remedy against it, people used to appeal to supernatural powers to be cured. In catholic countries, several saints were invoked against epilepsy and were therefore called *saints convulsionnaires* (convulsionary saints) in French. One of them was St Valentine. Indeed, he was considered the patron saint of people with epilepsy, and the illness was often called *mal St. Valentin* (St Valentine's disease) in French. The Germans used *St. Veltinskrankheit*, *St. Veltinsplage* (St Valentine's plague), or *St. Veltinsarbeit* (St Valentine's toil). A Polish representation of St Valentine has a caption that says *St Valentine, patron against the severe disease*. The saint is seen wearing the ritual garment of an exorcist (Figure 2.1).

In Dutch *sintvelten* became a synonym for 'epilepsy' as did *Sankt Veltin* in German. One could curse somebody out with the words *Ich wolt, dasz er Sanct Veltin het!* ('I wish he had St Valentine', i.e. epilepsy). The Dutch idiom *iemand naar Sint Velten wensen* means 'to call on fate to visit someone with Saint Valentine', i.e. 'to curse someone'.

Why was St Valentine invoked against epilepsy? According to some etymologists, the name of the Latin saint Valentinus, after it had become

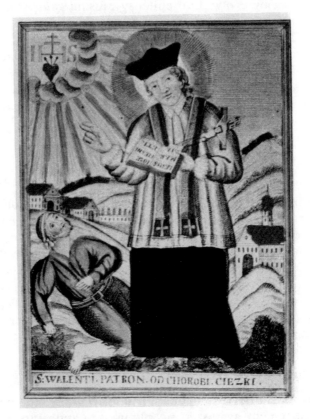

Figure 2.1: St. Valentine, patron against epilepsy.

Veltin – /feltin/ – in German, was equated to the homophonous phrase *fällt hin*, i.e. '(he) falls down'. Since falls were considered to be the main symptom of epilepsy, St Valentine came to be associated with the disease.

There is another possibility, however. The Latin name Valentinus became *Valtl* in Southern Germany. Due to a formal resemblance it was confused with *Veit* – /vait/ – which was the German name of another saint, Vitus, who used to be invoked against chorea, a disease which is also called *St Vitus's dance*. Since chorea was not always clearly distinguished from epilepsy and St Valtl was often confused with St Veit, the former saint came to be associated with chorea and with epilepsy.

At Rouffach (or Rufach) near Colmar in Alsatia, there was a church with a shrine containing relics of St Valentine. In the Middle Ages, Rouffach became a famous place of pilgrimage for sufferers from epilepsy. A hospital was built which accommodated the sick pilgrims. A woodcut from the time (Figure 2.2) represents St Valentine blessing devotees, two of whom are lying on the ground. A pig near St Valentine probably represents the devil whom the saint

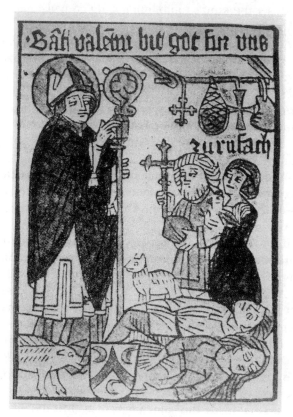

Figure 2.2: St Valentine venerated at Rouffach, France.

has exorcised. The German legend says *Sankt Valentin bit got für uns zu rufach* ('St Valentine, pray to God on our behalf at Rouffach').

As chorea was not clearly distinguished from motor seizures, St Vitus was at times prayed to regarding epilepsy, and was entreated to free the patients from the fiend who possessed them. Therefore, he was often represented with a cock, a bird which, according to ancient beliefs, could drive away evil spirits.

The confusion of epilepsy with chorea may explain why another saint, Willibrord, was invoked against epilepsy. Willibrord, an English monk, came to the continent and founded the monastery of Echternach (now in the Grand Duchy of Luxemburg). In the thirteenth century, the city of Echternach was plagued with dancing mania, a hysterical disease sometimes confused with St Vitus's dance. The inhabitants prayed to St Willibrord to be delivered from the epidemic. Their prayers were answered and St Willibrord was considered a protector against chorea and hence against epilepsy.

According to another tradition, people with epilepsy used to come and dance frantically by the saint's tomb, mimicking convulsions or chorea. The purpose was to be cured of either disease through imitative magic: *similia similibus curantur* (the like heal the like). The well-known dancing procession of Echternach is supposed to have originated from this practice.

St Lupus was another patron saint against epilepsy. The disease therefore was sometimes called *morbus St. Lupi* or *morbus Beati Lupi* in Latin, and *mal (de) Saint Loup* or *mal Saint Leu* in French. One legend has it that someone misbehaved at the burial of the saint and therefore was stricken with epilepsy. Eventually he repented and was cured. According to another tradition, St Lupus once destroyed a pagan idol. The priest of the idol tried to kill the saint in revenge but was instantaneously stricken with convulsions. Yet another explanation is that no demon could resist St Lupus. Accordingly, the saint was called upon to drive out the evil spirits supposed to possess people with epilepsy.

St Mathurin (or Matelin) of Larchant, France, was also said to have been a powerful exorcist and was therefore prayed to in cases of epilepsy. He was often represented blessing a patient out of whose mouth or skull a small demon was escaping. All around the saint were fetters symbolizing possession.

St John the Baptist was another saint often invoked against the disease, which for that reason was called *mal Saint-Jean* in French, *Gehanskränkt* (Johannes' or John's disease) in Luxembourgian, and *sint-janseuvel* or *sint-jansplaag* in Dutch. People suffering from epilepsy used to pilgrimage to the cathedral of Amiens in northern France, where a skull supposed to be St John's is preserved.

It is not clear what made this saint a patron against the illness. A tradition has grown up that he himself was afflicted with epilepsy. According to others, when St John was decapitated, his head fell to the ground. As patients with grand mal seizures also fall to the ground, the similarity between the saint's fate and the patients' involuntary behaviour led to the saint being invoked against epilepsy. Although it has been endorsed by some authorities, including the French physician Ambroise Paré (1517–1590), this explanation is less than convincing.

Like Valentine and Willibrord, John the Baptist was also associated with chorea. He was therefore sometimes called a *dancing saint* and some of the churches dedicated to him were visited by dancing pilgrims.

In Germanic countries, yet another saint used to be called upon to assist in case of epilepsy or to protect one from the disease: St Cornelius. The illness therefore is sometimes called *sint-cornelisziekte* in Dutch.

In Belgium, until recently, children were often given four names at birth. The first name was the one normally used to call the child. The second and third names were generally the first names of the child's godfather and godmother, or of the child's grandfathers or grandmothers. Not infrequently in the northern (i.e. Dutch-speaking) part of Belgium the fourth name was *Corneli(u)s* (or its feminine form *Cornelia*). By giving their child the name of the saint, parents sought to protect it from epilepsy.

In some places in Flanders parents would offer St Cornelius a quantity of cereal equal to the weight of their child to secure the saint's protection against epilepsy. This practice was called *counterpoising* or *counter-weighing*.

In Soignes Forest near Brussels there is a small chapel dedicated to St Cornelius. A plaque affixed to the front of the chapel says (in Dutch) *St Cornelius, pope and martyr, patron against cramp, paralysis and epilepsy* (Figure 2.3). The last three words in this caption were often used synonymously. Indeed, epilepsy was at times confused with several other diseases causing cramps, convulsions and/or paralysis.

One of the conditions that were not always adequately distinguished from epilepsy is *ergotism*. This is a very severe and often fatal illness caused by fungi (claviceps purpurea) found in rye and other cereals. Ergotism may take on different forms, one of which includes cramps and convulsions reminiscent of epilepsy. This form used to be called *convulsion céréale* (convulsions caused by cereals) in French.

Another form of ergotism is characterized by burning pains in the extremities which eventually become gangrenous due to contraction of the small arteries. Because of the 'ardent' pains it caused, the disease was often called *ignis ardens* or *ignis sacer*. The French spoke of *mal des ardents* (ardent disease), *feu sacré* (sacred fire) or *feu infernal* (hell's fire). These various names were also used to refer to herpes zoster (also called *shingles*) and to erysipelas, two diseases which may also cause burning pains.

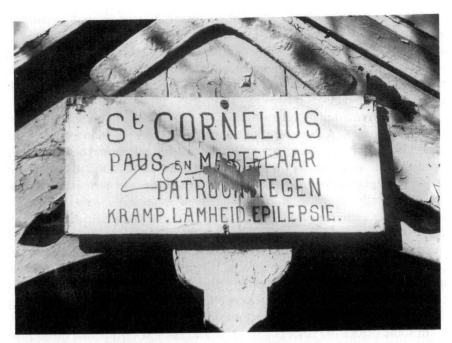

Figure 2.3: St. Cornelius, patron against epilepsy.

St Anthony used to be invoked against the ardent disease, which for that reason was frequently called *St Anthony's fire*. Due to the confusion between ergotism and epilepsy, the saint was occasionally also invoked against epilepsy. Conversely, St Cornelius was sometimes prayed to by those suffering from convulsive ergotism. Hence it was that *St Cornelius's disease* could refer to epilepsy as well as to ergotismus convulsivus.

Not only St Cornelius's but also St Ghislain's protection used to be besought against epilepsy, which was therefore sometimes called *mal (de) Saint-Ghislain* in French. St Ghislain founded a monastery in the southern part of Belgium, near a town which now bears his name. The monastery enjoyed great fame until the eighteenth century, but it was pulled down in 1797 during the French occupation. In the town of Saint-Ghislain, there was a church dedicated to St Martin which had an altar consecrated to St Ghislain. Children suffering from epilepsy would be brought to this altar in the hope that they might be healed. Many parents would put a necklace with a medal bearing the effigy of the saint around the neck of their newborns in order to protect them against convulsions.

The youngest son of King Philip IV of Spain (seventeenth century) died of a disease thought to be epilepsy. Because he was afraid that his eldest son might fall a victim to the same illness, the king had a small piece of Saint

Ghislain's relics, which were preserved in the Belgian monastery, sent to Madrid.

Not infrequently in South Belgium the fourth name given to boys was *Ghislain*. For girls, the feminine form of the name, *Ghislaine*, was used. As was the case with *Corneli(u)s*, parents hoped in this way to protect their children from the disease.

In southern Belgium yet another saint would be supplicated in case of epilepsy: St Giles, whose Latin name was Aegidius. In Walloon dialects the illness was therefore referred to as *l(i) ma* or *mau (di) sint djîle* (St Giles's sickness). Although he was very popular in the Middle Ages, little is known about St Giles. He apparently lived as an eremite in southern France in the seventh century. Because he was associated with epilepsy, it was sometimes claimed that he was a brother of St Cornelius (although St Cornelius actually lived in the third century). Not infrequently he was prayed to together with St Valentine, St Vitus, St John the Baptist, and St Cornelius. These saints were thought to form a sort of spiritual fraternity which was much more powerful than each saint separately. Giles's day (the first of September) coincides with that of Saint Leu's and this may have contributed to making him a patron against epilepsy.

The three wise men who, according to Matthew (2:9-11), followed the star to Bethlehem and, when they saw the child with his mother Mary, fell on their knees, gave him presents and worshipped him, also used to be invoked against epilepsy. If their names, *Gaspar*, *Melchior* and *Balthasar*, were spoken into the ear of a patient during an attack, the attack would cease immediately, people said. By engraving the three names on a cramp-ring (see above) one could increase its healing power.

The wise men's names were also included in prayers and formulae written on slips of parchment. The slips were supposed to protect those who wore them, as the following example dating from the seventeenth century shows:

> Gasper with his myrrh beganne
> these presents to unfold,
> Then Melchior brought in frankincense,
> and Balthasar brought in gold.
> Now he that of these holie kings
> the names about shall beare,
> The falling yll by grace of Christ
> shall never need to feare.

To be really efficient, the formula had to be written with blood. In fact, blood – especially from a fresh wound – had from time immemorial been considered a remedy against epilepsy. In Rome, patients would drink the blood of slaughtered gladiators. In the Middle Ages, the mouth of patients having a seizure was sometimes smeared with blood in an effort to end the access.

Plants against epilepsy

Beside cheese-rennet (see above), a variety of other plants were thought to be efficacious against epilepsy. Mistletoe was one of them. It was particularly effective if it was collected from an oak at the new moon and if it did not touch the earth before being used. By drinking infusions of mistletoe that had not fallen to the ground the patient would be protected by sympathetic magic from losing consciousness and falling to the ground. At Isigny-le-Buat in Normandy (France) there used to be a venerable oak bearing mistletoe to which people suffering from epilepsy would pilgrimage to be relieved of their plague.

Popular medicine also recommended the dried rhizome and root of hellebore. It would seem that this plant was used primarily as an emetic or cathartic to rid the patient of the excess of phlegm thought to be responsible for the seizures (see above). The violet, the pansy and the lily-of-the-valley were also thought to purge the body of excessive fluids and were therefore used to eliminate the cause of epilepsy.

To prevent attacks it was advised to drink infusions of passiflora, poppy, valerian, vervain, or of flowers of a lime tree. These plants all have a recognized sedative influence on the nervous system and may therefore have been found to reduce the number or severity of seizures.

Decoctions of the dried root of butterbur (*petasites*) and of the blossoms of mugwort (*artemisia vulgaris*) were also used. The mugwort starts flowering around St John's day (24 June) and is therefore sometimes called *sint-janskruid* (St John's plant) in Dutch and *herbe de (la) Saint-Jean* in French. The association of the plant with a saint who used to be invoked against epilepsy (see above) may have contributed to the belief that the herb could remedy the disease. This may hold true in respect of St John's wort, a common wild plant called *hypericum* in Latin.

Pieces of coal found under or near the root of a mugwort on the eve of the day of St John were equally thought to be efficient against epilepsy.

Frankincense too was recommended, probably because of its association with the three wise men.

Draughts of peony root were also considered salutary. And some parents had their young children wear necklaces made of peony seeds or peony roots to avert convulsions. To be fully efficient, seeds and roots had to be collected on a moonless night. The peony was already used as an anticonvulsant by the ancient Greeks, who considered it the queen of the plants and dedicated it to Paeon, physician of the gods.

Necklaces made of juniper berries, cherrystones or walnuts were also used as talismans against epilepsy.

Metals against epilepsy

Not only plants, but also metals were sometimes held to be efficacious against epilepsy. People with epilepsy were advised to wear an iron crown in the hope that the metal would capture the disease and thus cure them.

In German, epilepsy, particularly as it affects children and causes convulsions, is sometimes called *Fraisen*. To protect themselves from epilepsy people used to carry *Fraisenkreuze*. These were metal pendants in the form of a cross (Kreuz) bearing the effigy of a patron saint of epilepsy. This effigy was called *Fraisenmännchen* (little convulsion man).

Not only iron but also mercury was used to avert epilepsy. Toddlers were sometimes made to wear a necklace to which a small tube containing mercury was attached. The metal was supposed to protect them from infantile convulsions. However, a number of physicians advised against the use of mercury, which, they thought, might trigger epileptic seizures. Their opinion was based in part on the observation that people infected with syphilis not infrequently developed epilepsy. As mercury was often used as a remedy for syphilis, they related the seizures to the metal.

The history of epilepsy

The various names that were given to epilepsy are telling. They recount the adventures of the concept, and reflect the many ideas, misconceptions and prejudices that were entertained about the nature and aetiology of the disease. They also tell of the patron saints who used to be invoked against it and recall some of its famous victims. In fact, the nomenclature of epilepsy is a record of the history of the illness, and it reads like a biography.

CHAPTER 3

Ictal verbal behaviour

During epileptic seizures without loss of consciousness, patients may be prevented from performing verbal activities which they would like or have been requested to perform, or they may in spite of themselves perform them inadequately. Conversely, they may become unwillingly active and exhibit totally unintentional verbal behaviour. Thus, the excessive or disorderly firing of a hyperexcitable population of neurones may entail the suppression, the alteration or the activation of linguistic functions. It may cause interference as well as excitation. In other words, paroxysmal neuronal discharges may bring on not only negative but also positive symptoms: they may hamper volitional verbal actions or, on the contrary, induce involuntary ones.

Negative symptoms

Speech arrest

During simple partial attacks the patient may be unable to speak. If this inability occurs in the absence of comprehension difficulties, the patient is said to have a *speech arrest*.

During a speech arrest, patients cannot express themselves orally. Attempts to speak result in unintelligible grunts. At the end of the spell, the ability to repeat someone's words may be recovered before the ability to speak spontaneously. If a question is put to patients during a speech arrest, they can generally remember it, and they will answer it when the arrest ceases. This means that usually patients' memories are not disturbed during the seizures.

If the abnormal bioelectrical activity does not interfere with voluntary motricity apart from speaking, patients can follow verbal instructions and also write, although they are unable to express themselves orally. They may even be able to move their tongues, jaws or lips spontaneously or on command. In such a case, the speech arrest consists of a selective inhibition of the innervation of the speech apparatus.

Speech arrests may occur whether the epileptic attack originates from the left or from the right cerebral hemisphere. They are presumably due to inhibition of the motor speech mechanisms by the wildly discharging neurones, since deactivation of the epileptic focus by means of a barbiturate (such as sodium amytal) injected into the carotid artery during the seizure may reinstate speech (Novelly and Lifrak 1985).

Dysarthria

In some cases, speech remains possible during ictal episodes, but articulation is impaired. A patient with this difficulty in pronouncing words is *dysarthric* (from Greek *dys-*, meaning 'disturbed', and *arthr-*, meaning 'articulation') In the course of a seizure dysarthria may alternate with speech arrest. It may be so pronounced that speech becomes unintelligible. Dysarthria may be concomitant with drooling.

Aphasia

During an epileptic fit the patient may have difficulty in using language to communicate. This temporary verbal impairment resembles the *aphasia* that can be observed as an enduring condition in a number of brain-damaged people.

Very often, chronic aphasia results from damage to the left cerebral hemisphere. Similarly, in most patients with paroxysmal aphasia, the EEG points to an epileptic focus in the left hemisphere. More often than not, the focus lies in the temporal lobe.

Motor aphasia

Patients may be able to speak during the epileptic fits but may have word-finding difficulties. The seizure, then, may bring on a kind of *anomia* (also called *amnesic aphasia*). It may also happen that patients find it hard to initiate speech, and oral-verbal output is sparse. Indeed, they may be completely mute or solely able to utter profanities.

Written production is equally impaired. In attempting to write, the patients may produce a letter and then perseverate it, or they may write only the beginning of words and be unable to complete them. Reading is also disturbed, and may even be completely impossible. Finally, there may be some speech comprehension difficulties. This form of aphasia is called *motor aphasia*.

Hécaen and Piercy (1956) noted that there are proportionally more left-handed than right-handed patients with epilepsy who evidence ictal motor aphasia. From this observation they concluded that in left-handed individuals language tends to be represented bilaterally in the brain, i.e. in left-handers the two hemispheres are more or less equally involved in language processing. This conclusion receives support from the finding that following acquired unilateral brain damage, aphasia is significantly more frequent in left-handed than in right-handed patients (Satz and Bullard-Bates 1981). Conversely, recovery from aphasia due to a cerebro-vascular accident is significantly better in patients with left-handed tendencies or with familial left-handedness than in strongly right-handed patients of right-handed stock (Subirana 1958). It would appear, then, that cerebral dominance for language is less pronounced in left-handed than in right-handed subjects.

Sensory aphasia

During an epileptic attack a patient may also evidence a language impairment resembling chronic *sensory aphasia*. In such a case, verbal comprehension is severely disturbed while speech production is copious but garbled. There may even be *jargonaphasia*, i.e. a verbal output replete with *paraphasias* (involuntary word substitutions), *perseverations* (unintentional replacements of adequate words by words used a little earlier), and *neologisms* (non-existent words produced unintentionally by the patient). However, the patient may be able to recite overlearned series or prayers (nearly) correctly.

Jargonaphasia may be accompanied by logorrhea, the patient being prolix in addition to producing deviant speech. Loquacity at times looks compulsive: it is as if the patient cannot stop talking.

In paroxysmal sensory aphasia, written production is equally disordered. Indeed, there may be *jargonagraphia*. Souques (1928) had a French-speaking patient who suffered from petit mal epilepsy. One day, she had an absence while she was writing a letter. The beginning of her letter was quite normal, making allowance for a few spelling errors due to her socio-cultural status (she was a maidservant). The second half of the letter, however, was full of neologisms, perseverations and paragraphias and was therefore largely unintelligible. The transition between normality and jargonagraphia was sudden: down to 'revenir tout d'un coup' (recover all of a sudden) the text was fully appropriate, but the rest was gibberish:

Paris, le 2O août 1920.

Chère Madame M . . .
Je vous prie de bien vouloir m'excuser d'avoir tarder à vous écrire mais avec les patrons on a jamais fini, et même dimanche toute la journée il faut y aller vu qu'ils parte en voyage pour 8 jours au bord de la mer.
 Chère Madame M . . . samedi soir nous avons eu la visite de Monsieur M . . . qui a été bien fatigué et qui était bien peiné de vous voir souffrante, mais ce qui lui réchauffait le coeur c'est de voir les bons soins dont vous étiez entourée, il faut

espérer que votre santé petit à petit va aller en s'améliorant, l'on sait bien que cela ne peut revenir tout d'un coup et sournans ils vous exesperer vous vous expéserions que toute l'outre vous pitre pour voir ainsi le petit que le petit le pésion que la petite la soeur l'eau nous leçons il faut esperions la cortrietere va bien et que vous êtes vous êtes encre bonne santé.

Chers parents, je vous remercions sons de vous avons souviens nos parents nous vous avons devons clutions de vos nouvelles je vous remercions mercions davoir d'avoir dat vous d'avions a davoir davons vous etrions davons enrions vous irons ce que vous donniez en derrière ou vous donnez lirez en vous orniez ayez de vous de vous etiez de vez en ayez en ayez envoyez en serviexuxez de seviez les lescexiyez et je vous echiez de mes parialez qui ont bien plaiyez enexez de tout plait ayez et je vous axez une bonne santé et surtout la bonne santé.

Je termine chere maman en vous embrassant de cour somrbulle et bonne santé et surtout une meilleure santé ainsi que Pierriotte Votre Pierre qui vous entre de la prepiétaire et une grosse à vous libre ainsi que la Piriotte.

Maria Pierre terrotte Pierre vous dit bien les jours et bons chantillons.

Maria Pierrotte

(Dear Mrs. M . . .

I apologize for writing to you so late but at my employers' I never stop working, I even had to work last Sunday, as they are going to the seaside for a week.

Dear Mrs. M . . . Saturday night we had the company of Mr . . . who was very tired and who was very sorry to find you ill, but he was pleased to see how well looked after you were, it is to be hoped that your health condition will improve gradually, as obviously one cannot recover all of a sudden and . . . [the rest of the letter is untranslatable as it is made up of perseverations, paragraphias and neologisms]

Another example of ictal jargonagraphia was published by Hughlings Jackson and reproduced by Taylor and Marsh (1980). The patient was a physician, Dr Meyers, who during a psychomotor seizure wrote the following medical note:

For the last few days his beginning is more difficult for his tenderness of speechlessness and quick power of talk light swollenness of feet last three days. For the last 18 mos years there has been some decided indefinite on R side in dress circle.

To judge by the reproduction of the note in Taylor and Marsh's paper, the patient used no neologism and did not make literal paragraphias, i.e. did not make involuntary letter substitutions. His note is made of English words correctly spelled, yet it makes no sense. It is a pure instance of what Hughlings Jackson used to call *word salad*.

It may be assumed that Souques' patient and Dr Meyers were unaware of their jargonagraphia when it occurred. Otherwise they would most probably have stopped writing. In fact, Hughlings Jackson's patient himself confirmed that when a complex seizure occurred while he was writing he had the feeling that his written production was meaningful, correct and quite appropriate: 'My impression at the time that I was writing was that the words and sense were quite reasonable, and that I had kept within very familiar and prudent limits of expression' (quoted in Taylor and Marsh 1980).

Are patients with ictal jargonaphasia similarly unconscious of the inadequacy of their oral-verbal output? Do they realize that their speech is deviant or are they confident that they speak intelligibly and 'within familiar and prudent limits of expression'? Since patients who have sensory aphasia during seizures usually recover their full linguistic competence when the attack is over, one can ask them how they felt while they were having the seizure. A patient of Alajouanine and Sabouraud (1960) who had ictal sensory aphasia explained that when she used language during a fit, she always knew what she wanted to say, but she did not know whether she was wording her thoughts correctly. 'Je ne sais pas ce que je dis' (I don't know what I say), she stated. However, when she said something that was meant to be serious and her speech partner laughed, she concluded that she must have been using wrong words: 'Je me rends compte que ça ne doit pas être correct, puisque les gens rient, mais (moi) je ne l'entends pas' (I realize that what I have been saying must be inappropriate, since people laugh, but I myself don't hear my errors).

When expressing herself in writing, the patient was equally unable to judge whether her written production was adequate or not. In reality she used jargon also when writing. On the other hand, this woman knew that she could not understand what she heard when she was having an attack. And this awareness was present during seizures. Remembering an ictus in the course of which she was spoken to by a female physician, she stated: 'Elle me disait des choses que je ne comprenais pas' (She was telling me things which I could not understand). Other patients with a similar comprehension disorder report that they had the impression that the people around them had suddenly started using a foreign language.

Partial awareness of his language impairment was also present in a patient described by Lecours and Joanette (1980). This man had ictal aphasia primarily of the sensory type. Throughout his paroxysmal episodes he was aware of his linguistic impairment. Specifically, he realized that he could not understand language. During a spell he would deliberately turn on his wireless or go through his mail to find out whether verbal comprehension was returning, indicating that the fit was drawing to an end.

The patient was also aware of the inadequacy of his verbal output during seizures and therefore purposely refrained from talking whenever possible. When he did speak, he sensed that what he was saying was inadequate but he did not know exactly what was deviant in his language. 'I know that certain words I say are not correct,' he explained, 'but I do not know which ones and I do not know how I pronounce them.' This Canadian patient was totally unaware of the fact that he would sometimes insert a short English idiom or catchphrase in his French-like jargon. He did not know, and was very surprised to hear from the investigators, that he had a predilection for a neologism - /tuware/ - which kept recurring from fit to fit.

On the other hand, the patient was well aware of the fact that he tended to recover his writing skills somewhat faster than his speaking skills, and he would spontaneously resort to paper and pencil rather than to speech if during the anticlimax of an epileptic attack he felt the need to communicate verbally.

These two patients, then, knew that they could not express themselves adequately during seizures but were unable to spot their verbal errors or deviations if they spoke during an epileptic spell. They could not monitor their speech during attacks.

The information provided by patients with paroxysmal sensory aphasia may throw some light on the vexed question of whether people with chronic sensory aphasia (also called *Wernicke's aphasia*) are or are not aware of their deviant verbal behaviour. Ever since Wernicke in 1874 provided the first description of sensory aphasia, opinions have diverged as to whether sensory aphasics realize that they have comprehension difficulties and that their verbal output is anomalous. Wernicke himself expressed the view that the patients are unaware of their linguistic impairment. This claim has been echoed by many aphasiologists down to the present time. However, some clinicians disagree: they maintain that sensory aphasics are conscious of their verbal disturbance.

To the extent that the brain condition of patients during an epileptic seizure may legitimately be compared with that of patients having chronic aphasia, it can be assumed, on the basis of evidence obtained from epilepsy cases, that people with permanent sensory aphasia suspect that their language behaviour is deviant. They probably realize that something must be wrong with their expressive use of language but they do not know exactly what. In other words, they are partially anosognosic: they have but a limited insight into their neurolinguistic condition.

Language shift

Sometimes during fits, epileptic polyglots suddenly change languages in the course of speaking: they utter one or a few sentences in a second language and then return to the language of conversation. The contents of the second language sentence(s) usually does not fit in with the topic under discussion. The patients are generally unaware of their sudden and involuntary language shift.

Such shifts were observed by Schwartz (1994) in a polyglot woman, who on electroencephalographic examination proved to have bilateral temporal lobe spikes. Apparently the patient evidenced no clinical symptoms other than unexpected changes of languages, of which she was unaware.

Stereotyped verbal response

It may also happen that during an epileptic episode a patient evidences stereotyped verbal behaviour in response to verbal stimuli. For instance, they may answer *Yes* indiscriminately to whatever question is put to them.

Global aphasia

Ictal aphasia may also be global. In such a case, patients are unable to produce and to understand language whether spoken or written. They may be conscious of their double inability.

During a seizure, global aphasia may be preceded or followed by motor or sensory aphasia. Indeed, a so-called *Syndromwandel*, i.e. a characteristic change in symptomatology, may occur within an ictal episode.

At times, patients fail to comprehend speech because the epileptic spell makes them deaf. If this deafness is accompanied by a speech arrest, and the ability to use written language is not examined, the patients may be misdiagnosed as having global aphasia or as being unresponsive to the environment.

Chronic aphasia and epilepsy

If in a patient cerebral damage causes permanent aphasia, and if this damage also brings on epileptic seizures, the severity of the chronic aphasia may increase during attacks.

Aphasic status epilepticus

At times, ictal aphasia lasts for several hours, occasionally even a few days. Simultaneous serial electroencephalograms show frequent epileptic discharges. Aphasia does not disappear in the intervals between the bursts. Presumably the frequency of the bioelectrical paroxysms is such that it prevents the restoration of a normal verbal situation inter-ictally. This severe condition is called *status epilepticus with aphasia* or *aphasic status epilepticus*. Sometimes the adjective *partial* is placed before *status* to emphasize that the patient does not lose consciousness. The severity of the aphasia may fluctuate during the prolonged spell.

If aphasia is the only clinical manifestation of the status epilepticus, it may be mistaken for a language disorder of vascular origin and the patient be suspected of having suffered a stroke. Only electroencephalography can reveal the epileptic nature of the verbal deficit. Ictal aphasia regularly coincides with abnormal bioelectrical activity in the EEG.

It may also happen that the patient presents not with constant aphasia but with a quick alternation of (near-) normal and aphasic periods. In such a case the successive aphasic episodes generally correlate with electroencephalographic disturbances.

Confabulation

Patients with partial epilepsy originating from the right hemisphere may at times produce confabulatory speech during attacks. Their discourse is syntactically correct and relatively coherent but it does not fit the situation, or contains obvious inaccuracies.

This type of ictal verbal behaviour is probably akin to *confabulation* as it is occasionally observed in patients with right brain damage. These patients may show a tendency to produce inappropriate or irrelevant speech. An instance of this peculiar condition has been reported by Guard et al. (1983). When asked to tell the well-known story of *Tom Thumb*, their French-speaking patient said:

> C'est autre chose, ça n'a rien à voir avec cela, il a sorti son paquet d'oseille; il a compté les sous comparativement avec ce qu'il avait avant dans la caisse (That's another story, it has nothing to do with that. He took out his stack of dough; he counted his coins, in relation to what he had before in the cash-box.)

This type of disorder may be considered a disturbance of pragmatics: language is used in accordance with phonological and grammatical rules, but is inadequate: it does not fit in with the speaking situation and therefore lacks communicative value.

Disturbance of graphomotricity

In the case of ictal jargonagraphia reported by Souques (1928) and mentioned above, the patient's graphomotricity was not altered during the epileptic fit. The absence disturbed language use, but did not disturb handwriting: despite the attack the letters remained regular and well-formed, and the lines of writing were horizontal and evenly spaced. Were it not for the strange words, the second part of the patient's written message would not have betokened an epileptic spell.

In other cases, however, the seizure impairs graphomotricity. Handwriting becomes erratic, with elongated or poorly formed letters, and the page may get smeared. The text produced may remain appropriate, however, with adequate words and correct syntax.

Transient cognitive impairment

In individuals with subclinical epilepsy in the alert state, electroencephalo-graphic recordings made during the performance of intellectual tasks, including verbal ones, have shown that the occurrence of paroxysmal discharges during test administration often interferes with the performance either by slowing it down or by making it less successful. In other words, subclinical paroxysms not infrequently entail transient cognitive impairment.

According to studies by Aarts et al. (1984) and Siebelink et al. (1988), tasks requiring the use of verbal short-term memory are particularly likely to be disturbed by coincident subclinical discharges, except when the latter remain confined to the right hemisphere in right-handed individuals. In addition, Kasteleijn-Nols Trenité et al. (1988) have found that in school-children subclinical discharges occurring during a reading-aloud test tend to increase reading speed as well as the number of reading errors.

It may therefore be assumed that a number of children who suffer from diurnal subclinical epilepsy are regularly prevented from making progress at school or when doing their homework. In adults with this type of epilepsy, professional efficiency is liable to be reduced if vocational activities require sustained intellectual work.

A case reported by Aarts et al. (1984) shows that diurnal subclinical epilepsy may be reflex in nature. In their patient, a competent librarian, a number of intellectual tasks triggered paroxysmal EEG discharges which then interfered with the performance of the tasks. If he was asked questions at that moment, he could not always answer them adequately. No epileptic discharges could be recorded outside the performance of the precipitating tasks, and no overt clinical seizures could ever be observed.

Positive symptoms

Epileptic seizures may not only interfere with deliberate verbal behaviour or prevent the patient from performing linguistically, they may also induce involuntary vocal or verbal actions, of which the patient may or may not be conscious.

Cries and noises

At the beginning of grand mal seizures, just prior to falling to the ground, patients not infrequently let out a yell, the so-called *initial epileptic cry*. This scream may frighten those present if they are not familiar with epileptic fits. The yell is probably due to the incipient tonic contraction of the expiratory and laryngeal muscles. Partial seizures with an epileptic focus in the frontal lobe (whether right or left) may also begin with a shout, whereas in West's syndrome a cry is sometimes heard at the end of spasms.

Ictal cries may at times be protracted and show modulations correlating with paroxysmal bursts in the EEG.

During seizures, patients may produce inarticulate sounds involuntarily. These may range from grunts and moans to whistles and shouts. Patients may also smack their lips repeatedly or form clicks with their tongue. Again, involuntary howling may combine with running, as a case reported by Marsh (1978) shows.

Vocalizations

Some patients produce a protracted or iterative vowel sound during fits. These involuntary vocalizations can be associated with an epileptic focus in either hemisphere. Not infrequently the focus lies in or near the supplementary motor area in the superior part of the mesial aspect of the frontal lobes.

Speech automatisms

During partial seizures patients may also unintentionally utter words. These involuntary verbal productions are called *speech automatisms*. The utterances consist at times of mumbled words or of expletives. The latter are called *paroxysmal coprolalias*. Occasionally, involuntary swearing is accompanied by compulsive moving about or running. For this rare clinical manifestation the phrase *cursing and cursive epilepsy* has been coined.

Palilalias

During seizures, patients may involuntarily repeat the same utterance a great number of times. The *palilalic* utterance may comprise a single syllable or a single word or, on the contrary, consist of a (well-formed) sentence.

In some cases, the sentence is first uttered intentionally, for instance in answer to a question, and is then involuntarily repeated. Such repetitions are called *provoked palilalias*. They may exhibit some variation, the initial, deliberately produced sentence undergoing slight alterations as it is being compulsively repeated. It may also happen that during a seizure a completely unintentional sentence is produced a (great) number of times in a row. Such repetitions are called *spontaneous palilalias*. Some patients have only spontaneous, and others only provoked palilalias. Still others show both types of palilalias.

At times, spontaneous palilalias consist of reiterated neologistic strings of phonemes. Now and then, slight to moderate phonemic differences are observed between successive repetitions: the neologisms are phonemically akin but not strictly identical. An example of such variation has been reproduced by Bell et al. (1990) who observed it in a young woman with partial seizures due to an arteriovenous malformation in the posterior part of the left temporal lobe:

> . . . terpredeen zemexedrededeen zemexeverdedeen zemexeverdedeen mexeverd-edeen mexeverdedeen emexeverdedeen emexeverdedeen emexeverdedeen exeverdedeen exeverdedeen exeverdedeen exeverdedeen exeverdedeen . . .

The occurrence of this type of palilalia may have contributed to the belief that glossolalia is due to epilepsy.

Glossolalia, or speaking in tongues, is a verbal behaviour consisting in the production of concatenations of phonemes which sound somewhat like words and sentences but in reality form only non-words. These concatenations are often iterative, being made up of groups of phonemes that are repeated over and over again, possibly with slight variations. Glossolalia is usually, though not exclusively, observed within religious contexts. Members of various sects are in the habit of producing unintelligible utterances during services or when being at their devotions. According to the circumstances, such ejaculations are considered personal prayers offered to God, who is supposed to be able to understand them, or as messages sent by the Holy Ghost to the community through the mouth of the glossolalic speakers. In this case it is important that the messages should be decoded afterwards by the speakers or by coreligionists, lest the divine messages be lost.

There is no indication that glossolalia correlates with paroxysmal brain discharges. Glossolalic believers have not been found to be more prone to epileptic seizures than believers who never speak in tongues. There is no reason, then, to think that glossolalia is due to epilepsy, even though ictal palilalias at times resemble glossolalic utterances. In all likelihood, glossolalia is a non-pathologic manifestation of religious excitement or enthusiasm. It could nevertheless be the case that glossolalia and spontaneous palilalias consisting of repetitive neologistic strings of phonemes are produced by the same cerebral structures, namely subcortical nuclei (Fabbro 1998; Lebrun 2001: 27–30, 96). In patients with epilepsy these nuclei seem to be disinhibited, i.e. freed from cortical control, as a consequence of the paroxysmal bioelectrical discharges, while in glossolalic believers they appear to be stimulated by centrencephalic structures which subserve emotional life and are usually, though maybe not quite correctly, referred to as the *limbic system*.

In some patients, spontaneous palilalias vary from fit to fit. They may at times be relatable to some event(s) in the patients' lives. In other patients, the palilalic behaviour remains remarkably constant from spell to spell. A Polish immigrant in England would invariably repeat the sentence 'I beg your pardon' several times in succession at the beginning of a psychomotor seizure. He would do so even if the seizure occurred in the middle of a Polish conversation. He was unaware of his stereotyped palilalia, but his wife, whenever she heard him repeat the sentence, knew he was having an attack (Serafetinides and Falconer 1963)

Palilalias may be produced clearly or be mumbled or slurred. Sometimes they trail off, the last repetitions being whispered or simply mouthed. They may last as long as the epileptic spell or stop before the end of it.

Occasionally, palilalias are produced in association with non-verbal automatisms. During psychomotor seizures a patient of Schmidt and Wilder

(1968: 31) would execute a pantomime of going to bed while repeating 'I am sleepy, I am sleepy.'

Some patients remain fully conscious during their palilalic spells, as is shown by their ability to follow verbal instructions (Botez and Wertheim 1959). Others seem to have impaired consciousness and not to be aware of their palilalic demeanour. Patients who are aware of their palilalias may try to suppress them. They may proffer the word 'Stop' or a similar word in their attempts to end the involuntary repetitions.

Occasionally, palilalias are mental: the patient formulates a thought inwardly and then hears the formulation repeated over and over again in his head. An epileptic male quoted by Kapur (1997: 222) reported that 'once when out for a walk, I went through the pedestrian's wicket gate at a level crossing and noticed that the spring was rather stiff. I said to myself, 'That spring is too stiff' and then my thoughts, so to speak, 'stuck', so I went on thinking 'that spring is too stiff', 'that spring is too stiff', as if my brain was a gramophone and the needle had stuck in the groove.'

Ictal palilalias may arise with seizures having their starting point in either hemisphere. The focus may be in the temporal lobe, or in the supplementary motor area of the frontal lobe.

Paligraphia

It may also happen that during a psychomotor fit the patient repeatedly writes a letter or draws a sign. A patient of Gastaut and Zifkin (1984) would paligraphically draw the figure 6 or the figure O on any flat surface within reach.

Spontaneous repetitive verbal behaviour

Whilst some epileptics always produce the same spontaneous palilalia during fits, a patient of Palmini et al. (1992) would often say to whomever was around 'I love you' and correctly attach the name of the person spoken to. He was not conscious of his ictal behaviour.

Some patients produce a sentence such as 'I don't know where I am' or 'I feel funny' at more or less regular intervals during the seizure.

Gelastic and dacrystic epilepsy

Shouts and words are not the only sounds involuntarily produced during epileptic fits. Patients at times laugh or cry. If patients evidence unmotivated laughing during seizures, they are said to suffer from *gelastic* epilepsy (from Greek *gela-*, laughter). If they cry without reason, they are considered to have *dacrystic* epilepsy (from Greek *dacry-*, tear).

Paroxysmal laughing is sometimes heard during nightly fits, when the patient is sleeping. On the other hand, gelastic seizures may at times be triggered off by genuine laughing due to merriness or amusement. Again, ictal laughing or giggling may be accompanied by a blank stare and dilated pupils. Occasionally ictal laughter is followed by an atonic episode which may cause a fall. Contact with the environment may or may not be lost during gelastic or dacrystic accesses.

In the course of a single seizure, speech automatisms may alternate with compulsive laughing or crying. A patient of Hurwitz et al. (1985) had partial seizures with ictal laughter and the stereotyped utterance 'I have it'.

Negative and positive symptoms

Speech automatisms may also alternate with speech arrests or global aphasia. Thus, positive and negative verbal symptoms may at times be observed in succession within a single fit. The patient may evidence a reduction in linguistic competence or performance (negative symptom) alternating with a compulsive, more or less repetitive vocal or verbal behaviour (positive symptom).

Writing automatisms

Joseph (1986) reported having observed two patients with writing automatisms. During some of their seizures, these patients would produce written sentences involuntarily. They knew that they were writing but could not help it. Nor could they control their written output. Unfortunately, Joseph did not publish samples of this compulsive writing. It is not known whether the written output was intelligible and coherent.

Verbal hallucinations

During complex partial seizures patients may have the impression that they hear voices or words. The same words may be heard over and over again. They may or may not make sense. They may be the same whenever patients have an auditory verbal hallucination, or be different each time. After the epileptic spell, patients may or may not be able to reproduce them. Or they may report that they heard people speak but could not understand what they were saying. They may also indicate that the words they heard were not spoken but sung.

If the hallucination takes place while patients are listening to someone, the hallucinated words may disturb the comprehension of the real words. Indeed, they may supplant the real words, patients becoming deaf to their interlocutor's speech or mistaking the hallucinated words for their interlocutor's.

It may also be the case that the hallucinated words are words that were actually said by the interlocutor. The patients hear them now over and over again and are unable to pay attention to the new sentences spoken by their speech partners.

Occasionally an auditory hallucination combines with a visual hallucination. A patient of Chesni (1966) always had the impression that she was addressed by an unknown woman wearing a beige suit who invariably told her that she should not worry, as it would soon be all over. Foote-Smith and Bayne (1991) have argued that Joan of Arc's visions may have been auditory-visual hallucinations caused by epilepsy (see also above, p. 17).

If patients are not aware that they are having a hallucination, they may start talking to the people they see and hear. Conversely, if they are aware of the delusional nature of what they see and hear and if the verbal hallucination is regularly followed by a generalized seizure (secondary generalization), they may come to recognize the hallucination as a forerunner or aura of a major attack.

Ictal hallucinations may also be visual. For instance, during seizures, patients may have the impression that they see numerals, as in a case described by Gastaut and Zifkin (1984). Such visual hallucinations are usually caused by an epileptic focus in either or in both of the occipital lobes.

Pre- and post-ictal verbal disturbances

In the period preceding a clinical seizure patients may already evidence some linguistic impairment. They may have difficulty in articulating words, and this dysarthria may be accompanied by swallowing difficulties. They may also have pre-ictal aphasia, either motor or sensory. Pre-ictal motor aphasia may be associated with a strong urge to communicate verbally: the patients fervently want to speak or write but find themselves unable to do so. A patient quoted by Kapur (1997: 221) reported that 'several times [prior to a seizure] I felt an urgent desire to speak to anyone who happened to be close by, whether I knew them or not; I did not know what words I wanted to say, so the result was an intense mental conflict.'

Generally patients are aware of their pre-ictal linguistic difficulties. Indeed, they often learn to recognize them as antecedent signs of a seizure.

Post-ictally, there may also be transient dysarthria or transient aphasia. The latter is not always easy to distinguish from the temporary mental confusion which is at times present after a seizure. Occasionally, post-ictal aphasia is of the anomic type. The patient does not make language errors but has word-finding difficulties. Access to their mental lexicon is temporarily impaired.

Post-ictal aphasia is generally observed only after a seizure originating from the left hemisphere. Patients may also be unable to speak whilst their other verbal functions appear unimpaired. They are then considered to have a post-ictal speech arrest.

Non-epileptic paroxysmal verbal behaviour

Epilepsy is not the only condition that can cause transient speech or language disorders. A number of other neurological conditions may equally entail temporary disturbances of verbal behaviour. These disturbances generally occur suddenly, tend to be of relatively short duration and may be repetitive. However, they are not due to abnormal discharges of hyperexcitable neurones. They are paroxysmal but not epileptic. They are mentioned here because they clinically resemble genuine ictal disorders. Indeed, they are occasionally mistaken for epileptic impairments of linguistic functions.

Paroxysmal dysarthria in multiple sclerosis

In patients with multiple sclerosis, active or expanding stages of the disease may be accompanied by short spells causing various transient cerebellar symptoms, including dysarthria. The latter may be so severe as to render speech unintelligible. Consciousness is not altered during the fleeting episodes, which usually last from a few seconds to a minute or two. Patients whose speech becomes difficult to understand may deliberately refrain from speaking. This voluntary silence should not be mistaken for a speech arrest.

The episodes may be ushered in by some dizziness or a sensation resembling a short aura. They occur spontaneously or when the patient is under emotional stress. They can generally be triggered off by hyperventilation. Usually they can be controlled with carbamazepine.

Between such bouts some patients are able to articulate normally. Other show a permanent dysarthria due to their progressive demyelinating disease. In these cases, paroxysmal dysarthria manifests itself as a sudden and short-lived aggravation of the chronic articulatory disorder.

Paroxysmal dysarthria in patients with multiple sclerosis does not correlate with anomalies in the EEG. No abnormal bioelectrical discharges can be detected during the episodes.

Speech arrests in Parkinson's disease

Parkinson patients may exhibit non-epileptic speech arrests. From time to time they suddenly become unable to activate their speech organs. They would like to communicate orally but are temporarily deprived of motor speech. During these episodes they may be unable to open their mouths on request, to chew, and to swallow their saliva, which then drips out of their mouths (*sialorrhea*).

At times, however, only deliberate propositional speech is transiently suspended, while reciting by rote is still possible. Also, emotional verbal ejaculations such as exclamations or expletives may occasionally be heard during speech arrests.

These episodes of mutism do not correlate with EEG anomalies. Consciousness is preserved. The patients do not fall but they may be hypo-kinetic, i.e. move slowly and restrictedly.

Paroxysmal palilalias, echolalias and coprolalias in post-encephalitic Parkinsonism

In patients with post-encephalitic Parkinsonism, which is a specific form of Parkinsonism resulting from an epidemic viral infection of the brain, there may occur spasms of conjugate ocular muscles causing involuntary eye deviations. The attacks may last from a few seconds to hours. During these oculogyric seizures patients may unintentionally produce spontaneous palilalias or, if other people are present and if the patients attempt to communicate with them, they may repeat each of their sentences a great many times in sequence (van Bogaert 1934). They may also repeat the interlocutor's questions instead of answering them, that is to say, they may produce *echolalias*. Patients may also unintentionally utter profanities or let out yells. They are generally aware of this compulsive verbal behaviour and may repeatedly try to apologize for it (Wohlfart et al. 1961).

Paroxysmal mental palilalias

Some Parkinson patients experience mental palilalias: they involuntarily keep repeating a word or sentence inwardly. During such spells they may be unable to perform deliberate actions (van Bogaert 1934).

Paroxysmal verbal disturbances in migrainous patients

Attacks of migraine may be accompanied or preceded by various verbal impairments, called *verbal accompaniments of migraine*. Aphasia may be such an accompaniment. A patient who used to have recurrent headaches associated with motor aphasia reported that she was always aware of her speech errors but could not avoid nor correct them:

> I could immediately recognize phonemic paraphasias. I did not have to infer from the listener that I was making mistakes. I heard the errors literally as they were happening. I was definitely conscious of what I wanted to say, but what came out in my speech was different from my intent. The sensation I had was that there was some intermediary between my conscious intent to speak a certain phrase or sentence and the production of the phrase or sentence – as if some alien force were twisting my words or saying what I wanted to say in a different way than I had formu-lated it in my mind. I did attempt to correct my errors after making them. Most of the time I could not . . . My attempts at self-correction were also fully self-conscious.

At times, patients experience marked word-finding difficulties during migraine attacks or just prior to them. As a result, their speech is slow, hesitant, and circumlocutory, but the words that they manage to produce are usually adequately formed.

There may also be migrainous episodes during which verbal comprehension is disturbed. The patients fail to understand what they are told or what they read. This impairment may be concomitant with fluent jargonaphasia.

In rare cases, migraine is accompanied by global aphasia. Patients are unable to use language during part or whole of migrainous attacks.

At times, only reading is affected. Patients have *pure alexia*. They can still write, but cannot read, not even what they themselves have written, as cases reported by Bingley and Sharp (1983) and Fleishman et al. (1983) show.

Attacks of migraine may also be accompanied by dysarthria or by a speech arrest: though not aphasic, patients are temporarily unable to articulate correctly; indeed, they may be completely unable to form words.

Dysarthria may also be a forerunner of a migrainous spell, and so may verbal hallucinations. Before headaches begin patients may have the impression that people around them are talking unusually fast.

Occasionally, migrainous patients experience spells of aphasia that are not accompanied or followed by headache.

Aphasia due to transient ischemic attacks

Vascular diseases or vascular malformations may cause transient ischemic attacks, i.e. temporary reductions of blood supply to some part(s) of the brain. These transitory disorders of the cerebral circulation may entail various symptoms including aphasia, which may be of the anomic type.

Paroxysmal dysarthria or mutism caused by neuroleptics

Patients treated with neuroleptics, i.e. drugs that modify the biochemistry of the brain, particularly of the centrencephalic structures, may have bouts of (severe) dysarthria or of mutism, especially at the beginning of treatment. In patients who have become comatose following an overdose of sedative or anti-depressant medication, temporary dysarthria is sometimes observed when consciousness is regained.

Spasmodic laughing and crying

In subjects with pseudo-bulbar palsy, i.e. with paralysis due to a (generally bilateral) hemispheric lesion affecting the motor corticobulbar pathways, there is often an impairment of the control over emotional reactions, as a result of which paroxysmal bouts of involuntary laughing or crying are observed. These bouts may be an exaggeration or prolongation of a normal affective response. Thus, patients laugh because they are amused, but having begun to laugh, are unable to stop.

The emotional response may also be totally inappropriate, as when the patient starts laughing on hearing bad news. In such a case there is a mismatch between the patient's overt reaction and his state of mind.

Finally, there may be bouts of completely unmotivated laughing or crying. These bouts may repeatedly interrupt deliberate speech (Figure 3.1).

None of these inadequate emotional behaviours, which are usually referred to as *emotional lability*, have an epileptic origin.

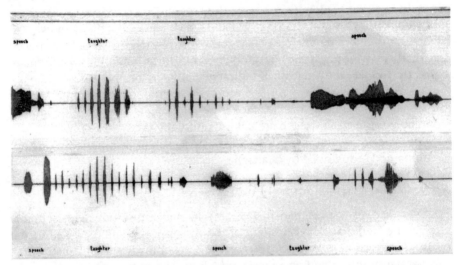

Figure 3.1: Bouts of involuntary laughing interrupting deliberate speech repeatedly.

Conclusion

Epileptic seizures may interfere with verbal behaviour, preventing the patients from performing linguistically as they wish or as would be desirable to ensure efficient communication. In some cases, they are totally unable to use language (paroxysmal global aphasia). In others, the command of language is impaired (paroxysmal motor or sensory aphasia). In still others, verbo-motor impulses are prevented from reaching the periphery (paroxysmal speech arrests) or do so inadequately (paroxysmal dysarthria, disorder of graphomotricity).

The abnormal neuronal discharges may also bring on unintentional verbal behaviours. The patient may involuntarily produce sounds or words or sentences. The latter may be compulsively repeated (paroxysmal palilalias).

While in some cases the patient always presents with the same ictal symptomatology, in other cases the symptoms are inconstant or even change from one attack to the next.

There is, then, a large variety of verbal behaviours that can be observed during partial seizures. Patients may preserve verbal functions during the fit, or they may lose them in part or completely, or they may exhibit an uncontrollable linguistic deportment of which they may or may not be conscious.

On the whole, negative symptoms occur more frequently than positive symptoms. Yet, they may alternate in the course of a single fit. Last but not least, the deviant verbal behaviour may be the only observable symptom during the whole attack.

Finally, there are neurological illnesses such as multiple sclerosis, Parkinsonism or migraine, which may bring on transient anomalies resembling ictal verbal behaviours. However, these anomalies do not correlate with pathological bursts in the EEG and therefore are not considered to be epileptic in nature.

CHAPTER 4

Language-induced reflex epilepsy

Reflex epilepsy is a variety of epilepsy that is regularly triggered off by a specific agent. In a number of cases the agent is a verbal activity. Reading, writing, speaking and listening to speech can all act as precipitants.

Reading epilepsy

By far the most frequently reported form of language-induced epilepsy is *reading epilepsy*. Reading, therefore, may very well be the most powerful epileptogenic verbal activity.

Seizures

Reading epilepsy consists of seizures induced by the act of reading. In some cases silent and oral reading are equally liable to provoke ictal episodes. In other cases, attacks are more likely to occur following oral than silent reading. In some patients, seizures are triggered off not only by reading texts but also by reading scores of music (e.g. while playing the piano). In a number of blind people, epileptic spells are precipitated by the action of deciphering Braille texts with the fingers.

The length of time during which patients can read before the attack begins varies not only from patient to patient but also from one day to the next.

Patients sometimes report that the epileptogenic power of reading is dependent on the nature of the reading material. However, their claims cannot always be confirmed medically or electroencephalographically. While examined in the clinic, these patients may fail to have a seizure although they are made to read the type of literature thought by them to be most epileptogenic.

The spells precipitated by reading may comprise observable signs or, on the contrary, remain subclinical. In the latter case, paroxysmal discharges are recorded in the electroencephalogram but no behavioural manifestation is noted.

Clinical seizures

The most frequent clinical manifestation of reading epilepsy is jaw jerking. The involuntary muscle contractions causing the jaw movements may be unilateral or bilateral. The jerks may be visible to an external observer or be simply felt by the patient. If they occur during oral reading, they may be accompanied by hesitant delivery or by stutter-like repetitions or blocks.

The mandibular twitches may occur together with a sensation of tightness in the throat, or of pressure in the head, or be accompanied by some dizziness. Instead of the jaw jerking or concomitant with it there may be eye blinking, involuntary movements of the extremities or muscular spasms. In addition, patients may experience a feeling of fear or of discomfort.

If the patient continues to read despite the unintentional muscle contractions, the partial motor seizure may evolve into a generalized seizure with loss of consciousness. At times, the seizure generalizes even if reading is interrupted as soon as the involuntary muscular contractions appear.

In other cases, the seizure does not generalize if reading is continued, but patients become confused or unable to understand what they are reading. In addition, they may have the impression that the letters move or are distorted in the text in front of them.

At times, the written comprehension disorder (alexia) occurs in the absence of muscular contractions. But it may be accompanied by some degree of aphasia, the patient's verbal output becoming laborious or paraphasic.

Unless the seizure generalizes, consciousness is usually preserved during a reading-induced attack. However, patients may involuntarily perform slight repetitive movements (automatisms) of which they are hardly aware.

If reading is interrupted when the first epileptic signs manifest themselves and if the signs then vanish, they tend to recur more quickly if reading is resumed a little later. Occasionally, reading induces absences or grand mal attacks not preceded by partial fits.

Seizures may sometimes be avoided by changing the usual pattern of reading. If patients susceptible to reflex paroxysms when reading are made to tap the table whenever they come across a word containing a specified letter, this unusual way of reading may render them (temporarily) immune to reading attacks.

Reading epilepsy usually begins in the second or third decade of life. It is rarely observed in schoolchildren learning to read. It affects males more frequently than females. More often than not, patients with reading epilepsy have first-degree relatives who suffer from one or another form of epilepsy.

Primary vs. secondary reading epilepsy

Some researchers distinguish between *primary* and *secondary* reading epilepsy. The former is a reflex epilepsy which is brought on exclusively by reading, whereas the latter can be triggered off by reading as well as by some other stimuli.

Patients with primary or secondary reading epilepsy may, in addition, show minor or major seizures whose starting mechanism is not known, i.e. seizures that do not appear reflex in nature and are therefore called *spontaneous*.

Interestingly, in patients with both reading and spontaneous epilepsy the occurrence of a reading-induced attack may for some time free them from non-reflex seizures. On the morning of her wedding day, a patient of Alajouanine et al. (1959) deliberately read until a reflex ictus occurred. She could then be pretty sure that no epileptic spell would disturb the wedding ceremony.

Reading epilepsy can be symptomatic or idiopathic: in some cases, a detectable cerebral damage can legitimately be considered responsible for the seizures, while in others no such damage can de discovered.

Priming

Reading may act not only as a trigger but also as a primer, that is to say, that it may facilitate the elicitation of reflex seizures by other stimuli. For instance, after having read for some time, patients may have subclinical paroxysmal discharges or experience involuntary muscular contractions if they then start speaking or writing. Reading may also render them light-sensitive. After he had been reading for a while a patient of Stevens (1957) had an epileptic fit precipitated by a sudden flash of light.

Electroencephalography

Electroencephalographic findings are heterogeneous in reading epilepsy. In some cases, recordings at rest are normal, and such provocative factors as sleep, hyperventilation, intermittent photic stimulation and visual pattern stimulation all fail to elicit pathological discharges. Bioelectrical anomalies are observed only during (oral) reading. They sometimes begin as soon as the patient starts reading and cease as soon as the patient stops reading. In other cases, spontaneous or provoked anomalous activity is recorded also when the patient is not reading.

During reading, discharges are sometimes registered over one and sometimes over both hemispheres. Bilateral discharges may be symmetrical and/or synchronous. When unilateral, they are generally lateralized to the left side of the brain. Paroxysmal discharges may correlate with the involuntary clonic or tonic muscle contractions.

Pathogenesis

It is still uncertain which features of the reading process trigger off the parox-ysmal brain activity. A number of researchers consider the eye movements to be the epileptogenic stimuli. Some of them incriminate the wide leftward gaze sweep at the end of each line of reading, while others assume that the quick, saccadic rightward eye movements precipitate the seizures.

Some clinicians are of the opinion that the alternations of black (words) and white (spaces) stretches on the written or printed page elicit attacks in much the same way as intermittent photic stimulation does.

These various views fail to account for the fact that, in blind patients, reading by touch may at times precipitate seizures. Obviously, in blind people, scanning eye movements or sensitivity to black-white alternations cannot be incriminated. Moreover, as regards the third hypothesis, it may be noted that in a number of seeing patients suffering from reading epilepsy, intermittent photic stimulation does not bring on pathological discharges.

Some experts implicate the articulatory movements that are performed during reading, whether these are overt as in oral reading or covert as in silent reading. In patients who have seizures following oral but not following silent reading, it is assumed that subliminal articulatory movements are too weak to cause abnormal bioelectrical discharges. Still other epileptologists regard the mental concentration required by reading as the chief determinant of the seizures.

This diversity of opinions shows that the pathogenesis of reading epilepsy is still poorly understood. It may actually be the case that reading epilepsy can be brought on by a variety of factors. The starting mechanism need not be the same in all patients. What the cause may be in each individual case remains a matter of conjecture.

Writing epilepsy

Not only reading but also writing can be epileptogenic, though to a lesser extent. It can cause absences as well as clonic or tonic muscular contrac-tions. For instance, the writing hand may jerk or freeze. In some cases, motor symptoms occur as soon as the patient starts writing. They may be such as to prevent them from even signing their name. Motor symptoms may also be ushered in by a hallucination. For instance, patients may suddenly have the impression that the letters they have just written rise from the page.

Changing the usual writing pattern may or may not be effective in averting seizures. Some, but not all, patients are seizure-free when they write with their non-preferred hand.

Like reading epilepsy, graphogenic epilepsy may be primary or secondary. In patients with secondary writing epilepsy, reading not infrequently proves epileptogenic. In addition to their primary or secondary reflex attacks, some patients have spontaneous seizures.

As in reading epilepsy, electroencephalographic findings are not uniform. In some patients, the rest EEG is normal, in others it is pathological. In patients with normal rest EEG, provocative manoeuvres may or may not be effective in bringing on pathological discharges.

Other graphic activities

Patients suffering from writing epilepsy may be able to draw even for prolonged periods of time, or to doodle or type, without having any clinical or subclinical seizures. Conversely, there are people who can write without inconvenience but in whom drawing or typewriting is liable to provoke seizures. There are also individuals who have attacks following written or mental calculation.

Drawing epilepsy, typing epilepsy and calculation epilepsy are usually secondary, that is to say, that other activities may also bring on seizures. These other incitants vary from patient to patient.

Playing the piano or the organ

An activity that somewhat resembles typing is playing the piano or the organ. This activity too may be epileptogenic. In rare cases seizures are likely to occur only if a particular tune is played, as in a case reported by Sutherling et al. (1980)

Speaking epilepsy

Speaking epilepsy, i.e. epilepsy induced by speaking, seems to be rare. At any rate, there are few reports of seizures induced by speech acts. In some of the reported instances, speaking was likely to trigger off a seizure only after reading had precipitated one. Once an attack had been elicited by reading, a patient of Geschwind and Sherwin (1967) was for a time liable to have a second fit if he started to speak or to write. During such 'primed' episodes, he had palatal and jaw jerks and was unable to speak. He remained fully conscious and could follow verbal instructions, though. Whispering was as effective as speaking loudly in triggering attacks. On the other hand, performing repetitive silent lip, tongue or jaw movements, humming a tune without words and drawing geometric forms did not provoke any seizure. The patient's rest and sleep EEGs did not evidence any abnormal bioelectrical activity, and intermittent photic or optokinetic stimulation failed to provoke paroxysms. During language-induced seizures, bilateral and symmetrical discharges could be recorded, primarily in the frontal regions.

A similar case was reported by Brooks and Jirauch (1971). If their patient started speaking or writing following an attack induced by reading, he was likely to experience jaw jerking. The jerks interfered with speaking, causing a sort of stutter.

There are also patients with reading epilepsy who occasionally have a speaking-induced seizure not preceded by an attack due to reading. Indeed, speaking epilepsy is sporadically observed in patients who cannot read. In a pre-schooler Herskowitz et al. (1984) noticed involuntary head and eyelid movements caused by humming, singing and recitation of nursery rhymes. The clinical signs were accompanied by bilateral bioelectrical discharges. On the other hand, conversational speech did not entail any unintentional movements or electrical paroxysms.

Finally, mention may also be made of Lee et al.'s description (1980) of a patient who had motor aphasia following neurosurgery on the left hemisphere. His attempts to speak, read or write regularly induced seizures without loss of consciousness.

Speech, then, may occasionally prove epileptogenic. However, in some cases, the patient's brain has to be sensitized by reading before speaking can induce an epileptic episode.

Listening-to-speech epilepsy

Epilepsy induced by listening to speech seems to be as rare as epilepsy provoked by speaking. As is the case with speaking, listening to speech is at times likely to elicit an attack only after reading has induced one. In other cases, listening to speech can trigger off fits although there is no reading epilepsy. Forster et al. (1969) have described a patient who had grand mal seizures, probably post-traumatic in nature, and partial seizures during which she would perform unintentional mouthing movements while being at the same time unable to speak. If holding something in her hand, she was likely to drop it. Post-ictally there was transient amnestic aphasia.

Most of these partial attacks occurred while she was listening to any of three different male radio announcers. Occasionally paroxysms were induced by other voices as well. The contents of the verbal messages seemed immaterial, as the reproduction by someone else of the sentences spoken by the announcers who induced epileptic fits failed to evoke any attack. Probably the patient's brain was abnormally tuned to some phonetic features of the three incitant voices.

The patient was hospitalized and progressive desensitization was attempted. She was made to listen repeatedly to tape recordings of the three announcers whose voices had triggered off epileptic fits. The tapes were presented regardless of the seizures they induced. After several days of sustained exposure the patient became insensitive to the noxious stimuli and could be discharged.

However, one day, she happened to listen to a new announcer, whose voice induced a seizure. As a consequence, she became sensitive again to the voices of the usual three broadcasters. The process of desensitization had to be repeated, this time involving four speakers. After a few days of frequent exposure to the incitant voices, the patient became seizure-free again.

A comparable case was observed by Ramani (1991). The patient had partial seizures, which were either spontaneous or reflex. Her reflex attacks included a feeling of pressure in the head, epigastric distress and mental confusion. They were induced by the sound of the voice of a female co-host on a popular television entertainment programme. If the patient watched the programme with the sound turned off, no seizure occurred. The EEG showed abnormal discharges in the right temporal lobe when the patient watched the programme with the sound present.

In a case reported by Tsuzuki and Kasuga (1978), ictal episodes were elicited by various auditory stimuli, including speech. Verbal messages in which the patient was interested were the most powerful precipitants. No clinical signs could be observed and no abnormal discharges detected when the patient spoke, although in all likelihood she was hearing herself. Furthermore, auditory stimuli tended to remain ineffective when she was engaged in an activity requiring her attention. Apparently, her brain was unusually sensitive to auditory perceptions that were of particular relevance to her.

Mention may be made here of a self-observation by Dr Myers, the nineteenth century physician who suffered from temporal lobe epilepsy (quoted in Chapter 3). Myers noted that during complex partial seizures he often had a feeling 'of sudden recollection of a forgotten fact', i.e. an impression of déjà vu. 'The recollection,' Myers added, 'is always started by another person's voice, or by my own verbalized thought, or by what I am reading and mentally verbalize.' According to Myers, then, the impressions of déjà vu that he experienced during some complex partial seizures could be induced by a partner's voice or by his own internal speech. Listening to somebody's words or to his own verbalized thoughts could bring on ictal phenomena.

Listening-to-speech epilepsy is a specific form of sonogenic or audiogenic epilepsy, in that it is elicited by a particular type of auditory stimulus: speech or voice. It may be compared with another form of sonogenic epilepsy, music(ogenic) epilepsy. Some patients with the latter form of reflex epilepsy are liable to have seizures when they hear music of any kind, and therefore often develop a fear of music or *musicophobia*. Others are sensitive only to a particular sort of music, e.g. classical orchestral music, or to a particular piece of music, or to the sound of a particular music instrument.

However, if a particular sound elicits pleasurable psychic seizures (see above, p. 5), patients may come to expose themselves deliberately to the triggering stimulus. Foote-Smith and Bayne (1991) have submitted that Joan of Arc's divine visions were auditory-visual hallucinations primarily provoked by the sound of church bells, which the young woman readily listened to.

While it can precipitate attacks in some patients, listening to speech may at times avert spontaneous paroxysms in others. As a matter of fact, some patients report that if they force themselves to listen attentively to a speaker when they experience an aura, they can often prevent the actual seizure from taking place.

Conclusions

Reading, writing, speaking and listening to speech can all precipitate epileptic fits. Of the four verbal activities, reading appears to have the greatest epileptogenic power.

The seizures induced by language may range from simple absences to partial motor fits to generalized attacks with convulsions and loss of consciousness. The partial seizures may be accompanied by confusion, comprehension difficulties or suspension of speech.

At times, however, the ictal episodes remain subclinical. Abnormal discharges are recorded electroencephalographically but no change is observed in the patient's behaviour.

Some people with language-induced epilepsy have spontaneous seizures in addition. Others have ictal episodes only when performing a specific linguistic activity. In still others, reflex fits can be triggered off by several incitants, including language.

The aetiology of language-induced reflex epilepsy has not yet been discovered. Various hypotheses have been propounded, especially as regards the pathogenesis of reading epilepsy, but none of them has been confirmed. Maybe the starting mechanism of seizures triggered off by language is different in different patients.

CHAPTER 5

Stuttering and epilepsy

Throughout the last century the view was repeatedly expressed that stuttering and epilepsy are (often) interrelated. For instance, in 1905, Féré stated that epilepsy is frequently associated with stuttering: the latter can occur during an epileptic aura or as an ictal or post-ictal verbal behaviour; at times, it is the sole clinical manifestation of a seizure. In 1953, Bolin contended that stuttering is a diagnostic sign of epilepsy. In 1958, West submitted that severe stuttering in children is in fact a special form of pyknolepsy (see above, p. 6). And Damsté (1990: 13) claimed that cluttering, i.e. precipitous and indistinct articulation, is frequent in children with epilepsy and may easily evolve into stuttering.

Is there any evidence supporting the opinion that stuttering and epilepsy are interrelated at least in a number of cases? The answer to this question is in the affirmative. However, the available evidence indicates that the relationship that may obtain between the two afflictions is not always straightforward.

Prevalence of stuttering among people with epilepsy

According to van Riper (1971: 49, 79), Harrison in 1947 and Gens in 1951 found greater prevalence of stuttering among patients with epilepsy than in the general population, while Berry in 1938 noted that epilepsy was more frequently encountered among children with stuttering than among children without stuttering. These findings suggest a link between stuttering and epilepsy but do not enable one to specify the nature of the link.

Stuttering in reflex epilepsy

As was noted in the previous chapter, in people suffering from reading or speaking epilepsy the paroxysmal jaw jerks may be concomitant with stutter-like repetitions or blocks. These dysfluencies may conceivably be brought on by the abnormal neuronal activity which causes the jaw jerk or, on the contrary, may result from the mandibular tremulation itself. In other words, stuttering appears in such cases to be a direct or an indirect consequence of epilepsy.

Interestingly, after the seizure, the dysfluencies may transfer to spontaneous speech and persist for as long as a day (Brooks and Jirauch 1971). Thus, in a number of cases, the reflex seizure seems to disturb cerebral speech production mechanisms, which then need some time to recover. Another possibility is that due to some memory or learning effect, the speech production mechanisms continue for a while to behave as they have been made to during the seizure.

Stuttering during or before spontaneous seizures

As was noted by Andermann (1987), there are patients who occasionally stutter during spontaneous seizures. Indeed, stuttering may at times be the only clinical manifestation of the episode. In such cases, the speech impediment seems to result directly from the abnormal bioelectrical activity of the brain. It is a negative ictal symptom just as speech arrests, dysarthria and aphasia may be (see above, pp 29–34).

Chronic stuttering in patients with epilepsy

A left-handed patient of Guillaume et al. (1957) had motor seizures and absences as well as permanent stuttering consisting of many blocks interrupting speech delivery. The rest EEG revealed an epileptogenic focus in the right temporal lobe. Electroencephalographic recordings during speech showed bursts of bilateral rhythmic slow waves in the fronto-temporal area. Following resection of the lateral aspect of the right temporal cortex, seizures abated and speech delivery became fluent.

In this case, the speech impediment appears to have been closely linked to, and possibly to have been caused by, the abnormal bioelectrical activity of the right temporal cortex. In other words, epilepsy and stuttering seem to have been causally related.

A patient of Mazars et al. (1970) had developmental tonic stuttering affecting conversational speech while sparing imitative and serial speech as well as singing. This patient had never had epileptic seizures. The rest EEG showed no anomalies. Depth electrodes recorded abnormal electrical bursts in the right temporal lobe during conversational speech. The bursts tended to coincide with the blocks in verbal output. Partial resection of the right temporal cortex resulted in durable improvement of speech delivery. In this case it looks as if activation of a number of neuronal circuits in order to produce conversational speech elicited pathological discharges in the right temporal lobe. The discharges interfered with speech delivery.

A patient of Terzano et al. (1983) presented with partial motor seizures as well as with a stutter consisting of blocks and iterations occurring at the beginning of conversational utterances. Imitative speech was not affected. The dysfluencies were accompanied by blinking and transient impairment of consciousness. The rest EEG showed diffuse paroxysms as well as polyspike paroxysms following spontaneous blinks. EEG recordings during conversational speech evidenced epileptic discharges which generally coincided with the dysfluencies in speech production. Treatment with valproid acid resulted in the disappearance of the seizures and the normalization of speech delivery.

Terzano et al. hypothesized that in their patient the desire to use speech conversationally induced involuntary blinking. The repeated eye closures elicited epileptic paroxysms which in turn interfered with speech production. Blinking reflex epilepsy, then, was responsible for the stutter.

Stuttering and epilepsy following brain damage

Following brain trauma. adults may present with stuttering and epilepsy. The two deficits may appear several years after the trauma and do not always begin simultaneously. Stuttering may be preceded by transient mutism and may manifest itself only episodically. As for epilepsy, it may be clinical or remain subclinical.

In some cases, anticonvulsants reduce the number of seizures and, at the same time, improve fluency. When this is so, it may be assumed that stuttering is the consequence of epilepsy: the abnormal bioelectrical discharges interfere with speech functions; their elimination or marked reduction through medication enables speech delivery to normalize. In other cases, when medication fails to improve fluency though it reduces the number and/or the severity of the seizures, there seems to be no causal link between epilepsy and stuttering; the two deficits are concomitants resulting directly from the brain damage that the patient has suffered.

The notion that post-traumatic epilepsy and post-traumatic stuttering may be relatively independent of one another is confirmed by the observation that one may occur without the other, or one may clear up while the other remains.

Stuttering and epilepsy following brain intoxication

Stuttering and epilepsy may be consequent not only upon brain trauma but also upon brain intoxication. Following chronic haemodialysis, patients may develop progressive encephalopathy with stuttering and epilepsy consisting mainly in myoclonic or grand mal seizures (Rosenbek et al. 1975). The stutter may be intermittent and may alternate with periods of mutism. It may be so severe as to give the impression that the patient 'is gagging on his words' (Madison et al. 1977).

Epilepsy and stuttering have also been observed following copper intoxication of the brain in patients with Wilson's disease, i.e. hepato-lenticular degeneration (Capon et al. 1973).

In such cases, it is not clear whether epilepsy is responsible for the stutter or is simply concomitant with it. Does the abnormal bioelectrical activity interfere with speech production, or do epilepsy and stuttering result directly from the damage suffered by the central nervous system? If no bioelectrical paroxysms can be recorded during speech, it may be presumed that stuttering is relatively independent of epilepsy. Another possibility, though, is that epilepsy has permanently damaged a number of neuronal circuits necessary for fluent speech. Speech delivery is then halting even if it is not concomitant with paroxysmal discharges.

Stuttering following anticonvulsant medication

A right-handed patient of Guillaume et al. (1957) had a severe developmental tonic stutter accompanied at times by involuntary foot or finger movements. Though he had never had clinical seizures and the EEG failed to reveal any paroxysmal bioelectrical activity, this man was given primidone. With this anticonvulsant a significant improvement of fluency could be obtained.

On the other hand, several cases have been reported in which administration of phenytoin to combat epilepsy brought on stuttering (e.g. Helm et al., 1980; Baratz and Mesulam, 1981; McClean and McLean, 1985). Reduction of the iatrogenic stutter could be achieved either by substituting carbamazepine for phenytoin (McClean and McLean, 1985) or by combining a small dose of phenytoin with a higher dose of carbamazepine (Baratz and Mesulam, 1981). It appears, then, that phenytoin, a well-known anticonvulsant, is liable to cause stuttering. The mechanism of this undesirable side-effect remains to be discovered.

Temporary disappearance of stuttering following an epileptic seizure

Manders and Bastijns (1988) have reported the intriguing case of a young boy with subclinical epilepsy and developmental stuttering. One day the child had a short partial epileptic attack followed by transient paralysis of the left arm (Todd's paralysis: see above, p. 3). When he recovered from the seizure, it was found that his stutter, which was rather severe, had completely vanished. It did not reappear until a few months later. In the meantime the boy had spoken fluently.

Can the temporary improvement of speech delivery following a partial seizure be accounted for? Can a plausible explanation be put forward for the influence that the epileptic access seems to have had on the stutter in the case reported by Manders and Bastijns? The answer to this question is in the affirmative. As a matter of fact, evidence is accruing that stuttering is due to insufficient or inadequate neocortical control over subcortical nuclei, particularly the basal ganglia, during (conversational) speech production (Lebrun 1997a, 1997b). As a consequence, any modification of the relationships between the neocortex and subcortical structures may conceivably have an influence on (conversational) speech delivery. The change may be brought about by disease as well as by surgery. For instance, Miller (1985) observed cessation of chronic stuttering in an adult with progressive multiple sclerosis, while Jones (1966) noted the disappearance of stuttering in a number of patients who had undergone neurosurgery because of a cerebral tumour or cerebral aneurysm. In the left-handed patient of Guillaume et al. (1957) and in the patient of Mazars et al. (1970) mentioned above, the pathological discharges originating in the right temporal lobe during speech probably interfered with neocortical control over subcortical nuclei. Resection of the epileptogenic focus was followed by a normalization of neocortical activity and, as a consequence, the disappearance of the stutter. A similar effect may at times be achieved with anticonvulsant drugs. By reducing or eliminating the abnormal bioelectrical paroxysms, the medication brings on an improvement of neocortical functioning and, consequently, of fluency. In the case reported by Manders and Bastijns, the clinical seizure may conceivably have caused a temporary change in the cortico–subcortical relations, which resulted in the temporary disappearance of the stutter.

Conclusions

As may be seen, the relationships between stuttering and epilepsy are rather complex. In some cases, the latter seems to be the cause of the former. In other cases, it looks as if there is no causal link between the two: they are simply concomitants, with, possibly, a common origin. Very occasionally, epilepsy, by modifying the relations between the neocortex and the subcortical structures, has a temporary beneficial influence on stuttering.

CHAPTER 6
Inter-ictal verbal behaviour

A number of patients with epilepsy evidence language or speech disorders only during seizures; between attacks their verbal behaviour is inconspicuous. Other patients show permanent verbal peculiarities or impairments; when observed or tested between seizures, their linguistic performances appear deviant or below norm

The aetiology of these *inter-ictal* verbal anomalies and deficits is often difficult to ascertain. In patients with cerebral lesions, both the epilepsy and the linguistic disturbances may be the consequences of the cerebral damage. If this is the case, the abnormal bioelectrical activity and the verbal impairment have a common origin but are not causally related: the language disorder does not result directly from the bioelectric disorder. Nonetheless, it is conceivable that the repeated electrical upheavals of (some part of) the brain may aggravate the existing linguistic deficits. As a matter of fact, it has been observed that if epilepsy can be controlled through the administration of drugs, the verbal handicap more often than not diminishes. When this is the case, one may assume that epilepsy tended to increase the linguistic disorder consequent upon the lesion.

In individuals with idiopathic epilepsy the repeated bioelectrical perturbations, if they are not medically controlled, may in the long run cause an alteration of brain tissue or of brain connectivity, or the development of new epileptogenic foci (called *secondary* foci). This may in turn entail cognitive deficits including language impairment.

Conversely, chronic administration of anticonvulsants may slow down cerebral growth and functioning and thus result in linguistic underachievement. Indeed, a number of drugs that help reduce the number and severity of clinical seizures have been shown to increase subclinical epileptic activity. This increase may in turn reflect negatively on verbal performances.

Again, in patients who regularly fall to the floor, the falls may cause small brain traumas which will eventually result in language or speech disorders.

In a number of cases, epilepsy is concomitant with mental retardation. For instance, youngsters suffering from the *Lennox-Gastaut syndrome* have frequent seizures which are often resistant to anticonvulsant therapy. In addition, they generally evidence (progressive) mental deterioration. The latter includes linguistic underachievement. It is not clear, however, whether epilepsy is the cause of the cognitive deficits, or whether both have encephalopathy as their common origin.

It would appear, then, that when epilepsy and chronic language impairment co-occur, the relationship between the two disorders is often difficult to ascertain.

Developmental aphasia

When marked underdevelopment of linguistic skills is observed in a child in the absence of mental retardation, hearing deficits, obvious neurological impairments, severe emotional disturbances or environmental deprivation, a diagnosis of *developmental dysphasia* is generally made. Synonyms are *developmental aphasia*, *congenital aphasia*, *developmental language disorder* and *specific language impairment (SLI)*.

In some patients with developmental dysphasia, expressive difficulties predominate: patients can understand speech substantially better than they can express themselves verbally. Their condition is usually referred to as *developmental expressive dysphasia*. In other cases, receptive and expressive abilities are underdeveloped to a more or less similar extent. This condition is called *developmental receptive-expressive dysphasia* or *developmental mixed dysphasia*.

Developmental dysphasia is usually distinguished from *language delay*. The latter is a milder disorder of language acquisition. If treated early enough, it generally resolves before the age of 6. In developmental dysphasia, however, acquisition of written language is limited and in some cases even impossible.

A number of children suffering from epilepsy present with developmental aphasia. Some of these children have clinical epilepsy while in others epilepsy remains subclinical.

Children with developmental dysphasia and subclinical epilepsy can be divided into two groups. The first group is made up of children whose diurnal standard EEGs show paroxysmal anomalies. These anomalies generally increase during slow sleep. Slow sleep (also called *slow wave sleep*) is the non-REM (rapid eye movement) sleep and occupies 75 per cent of an adult's total sleeping time.

The second group of children with developmental dysphasia and subclinical epilepsy is larger and is composed of children whose diurnal standard EEGs are normal, while the EEGs recorded during slow sleep evidence epileptic activity. In some cases this activity occurs during over 60 per cent of the total slow sleep time. It is observed more frequently in children with mixed than in children with expressive dysphasia (Picard et al. 1998).

Recent research on sleep and memory (see e.g. Wilson and McNaughton 1994) suggests that slow sleep may be involved in the storage of data in long-term memory. Nocturnal epileptic activity therefore may be presumed to interfere with this memory process and thus to hamper language acquisition. This is why a number of clinicians, including Gordon et al. (1996) and Picard et al. (1998), recommend that anti-epileptic medication should be administered. Others, notably Ronen et al. (2000), are somewhat doubtful of the influence of anticonvulsants, particularly sodium valproate, on developmental language disorders.

Not all children suffering from developmental dysphasia are afflicted with epilepsy: in some of them no seizures are ever observed and no epileptic discharges can be recorded electrographically. According to a study by Kutschke et al. (1999), children with developmental dysphasia and subclinical epilepsy achieve lower scores on tests of grammatical agility than children with developmental dysphasia and no epilepsy. Furthermore, dyslalia, i.e. underdeveloped articulatory skills, tends to be more pronounced in the group of children with subclinical epilepsy than in the group of children without epilepsy.

Metalinguistic skills

Compared to normals, patients with an epileptogenic focus in the temporal lobe tend to achieve lower scores on such metalinguistic tests as naming on confrontation, reproducing a heard story or a heard series of unrelated words immediately or after some delay, interpreting ambiguous sentences, and generating lists of words belonging to a specified semantic category or beginning with a specified letter. The deficit is usually more pronounced when the focus is in the left than when it is in the right hemisphere (Marsh 1978; Mayeux et al. 1980; Martin et al. 1990).

Pre-schoolers with simple partial seizures originating from the left frontal lobe and with no mental retardation tend to achieve lower scores than healthy peers on tests probing comprehension of prepositions and of narratives, repetition skills, lexical diversity or grammatical production (Cohen and le Normand 1998).

Hypergraphia

A number of people with epilepsy evidence *hypergraphia* or *scribomania*, i.e. they write much more than would normally be expected in view of their occupation and socio-cultural level. In addition, their written production is often replete with repetitions and superfluous or even irrelevant details.

Repetitions in hypergraphia may consist of words or phrases that are used iteratively, or of ideas that are expressed repeatedly in different sentences or through different codes. For instance, a number, quantity or date may be expressed by means of letters and immediately thereafter be pleonastically repeated by means of figures. It may also happen that a notion or event is first described by means of written words and then rendered pictorially by means of one or several (often identical) sketches or drawings.

A number of hypergraphic patients write extensive autobiographical reports or keep very detailed diaries. Others produce long lists of items of food or furniture, or of friends and relatives, or of their likes and dislikes, or keep minute records of their seizures and symptoms. Still others write songs, poems, aphorisms or prayers, or produce scores of unconnected jottings. In some patients, the urge to write may be so strong that they always carry a pad and a pencil with them. Others use whatever surface is available when they feel a compulsive need to write.

Some hypergraphics use special writing styles, such as calligraphy or mirror-writing. Specific words may be carefully underlined, or written in block letters. At times, the composition appears ritualized, with certain words or phrases repeated at regular intervals as a refrain or leitmotiv, or written with a different ink.

Some patients readily show their written production on request; others are reluctant to do so.

Hypergraphia is not confined to educated subjects. It may also occur in semi-literates. The written production of these people is usually replete with spelling and grammatical errors.

Blumer and Benson (1975) have published the following excerpt from the regular notes of one of their patients. The excerpt is representative of the diffuseness of hypergraphia:

When we moved from an upstairs apartment to a first floor one (Dec. 1, 19--), the squirrels I feed night and morning followed right with us. The squirrels are very tame and cute. They would feed out of my wife's hands. While I watch the door for a man to pick her up for work while she got ready I would prop the screen door open about 4 inches and feed them from inside by opening the inside door about an inch. They would come through the screen door opening and feed as I gave them food through the crack in the inside door. They would sit on the door sill and eat it (most of the time). It was winter and this way I could feed them while inside. When I went walking I would prop the screen door open and place some food in a dish on the door sill and they would feed from that. One day I did not put the dish there, they had enough, and went walking. When I came back the screen door had not gone completely shut and they had chewed about one third of the door away. I repaired this with water putty and painted it. Then to teach them to stay away from I rubbed some Red Pepper on the repair with my finger. As I watched the next day one of them must have got into it. He just stood on the porch. You could see he was in awful pain, he quivered, cried and dripped from the mouth. It was awful to witness but they have not bothered the door since. The next day (June 5) I took a dish of peanuts out on the porch to feed them. They all acted normal until I saw one coming from the side to get in the dish. He upset it and I went to brush him away with my hand. As I did he gave me a good bite on the outside of the right hand at the little finger. I washed it good with soap and water and put on some Merthiolate. I have been taught to watch the animal. If it has Rabies it will die in 10 to 14 days giving time to start the Pasteur treatment. Also the further from the head the bite is the longer it takes. Rabies is a virus of the nerves following the nerves from the bite to the head where it is fatal.

Our squirrels are fed clean food and water. They do not get into any dead or rotten food. They all are as healthy as can be. Have a pretty coat and the cutest habits you would want to see. The litter they had this spring were the most domesticated I have ever seen. Wouldn't you fight anything you knew treated you like he was with red pepper? Squirrels are like other forms of life. One alone you can train and it will respond without any trouble. But when another one or two show on the scene they are always fighting each other and chasing each other from tbe source of food. Also one always wants to be a bully. You should hear them growl and chase each other away when more than one tries to feed from the same dish.

I was a little alarmed about the bite because we have some neighbors who are scared of any animal at all. All they can say is "you know they can give you Rabies." Knowing circumstances I managed to conquer my nerves for a month and the squirrel was here and healthy as ever. After 2 weeks I felt safe, free and my nerves were quiet again . . . August 12 a squirrel came to the door. I thought it was a meek one. I held a piece of Graham Cracker toward it. It looked at me and went for my hand as if to take the cracker. It ignored the cracker and bit my finger instead. This time it was the little finger of the left hand. Within 10 seconds the bottom of my stomach hurt. I got a headache and the base of my throat started to hurt and feel tight. As I write this it is bringing back memories and I can feel it again.

I stood it as long as I possibly could. The worry was making a wreck of me. Then I went to Dr. R. August 17. He is treating me as you did. Reassuring me it was my nerves. Proving my thoughts and worries wrong and in my own thoughts. He told me to increase my Valium to half a tablet at 8:00 a.m. and half at 4:00 p.m. He also told me something I had read and forget. The state is considered Rabies free. There has not been a case I think he said in 5 or 7 years. This program of having dogs injected to prevent Rabies is purely political to make money and keep a record of dogs for licensing. Now I remember reading that in the paper when they started the program a few years ago.

Also do not feed the squirrels by hand. Toss the food to them or put it on a plate for them. They are wild animals and while no Rabies has been reported for a long time they can chew you up bad then infection maybe. He also reminded me that Bats are the ones that are full of Rabies. This I knew from childhood. Now I feed the squirrels in a dish on the porch. No more by hand. I slowly got ahold of myself again.

In superiorly intelligent individuals, hypergraphia may result in the production of a great number of valuable books and articles. As an example, the Japanese scholar Kumagusu Minakata (1867–1941) may be quoted. He is the author of a huge compendium on fungi found in Japan as well as of over 1,500 scientific papers on botany, biology, folklore, theology and sexology (Murai et al. 1998). Interestingly, he kept a diary in which he recorded his epileptic attacks together with other personal events. When writing he tended to form minuscule letters in a compact space. This instance shows that in patients with a high IQ hypergraphia is sometimes sublimated into polygraphy.

Hypergraphia is usually associated with temporal lobe epilepsy. It seems to be more frequent when the epileptogenic focus is in the right than when it is in the left temporal lobe (Roberts et al. 1982). Postmortem study of Minakata's brain revealed right hippocampal atrophy. The hippocampus is an important part of the infero-mesial aspect of the temporal lobe.

A number of clinicians, notably Geschwind (see Waxman and Geschwind 1975; Geschwind 1984) have advocated the view that many patients with temporal lobe epilepsy present with hypergraphia and/or excessive drawing activity. In addition, they not infrequently evidence hyperreligiosity, i.e. an intensive concern with religious, philosophical or ethical issues. Some of them lay great emphasis on morality and proper behaviour, even though their conduct in everyday life is often far from being irreproachable.

It has been further contended that people with temporal lobe epilepsy often have hyposexuality, i.e. reduced libido and lack of interest in sexual activity. On the other hand, they are frequently quick-tempered, with a readiness to become angry on slight provocation. They also have a tendency to become embroiled in petty arguments.

Such are the inter-ictal personality traits that are taken by some to be characteristic of patients with temporal lobe epilepsy. These traits are sometimes generically referred to as *Geschwind's syndrome*.

Prolixity

Some patients afflicted with epilepsy tend to be prolix, particularly when a seizure is about to occur. They indulge in digressions, get bogged down with irrelevant details or lay undue emphasis on accessory features to the point of losing track of the main facts. In picture description tasks, they not infrequently produce lengthy circumstantial accounts and wearisome interpretations of what the pictures represent (Hoeppner et al. 1987).

Patients may also repeat themselves over and over again or be reluctant to allow conversations to end. They tend unduly to prolong interpersonal encounters. This excessive cohesion is sometimes called *viscosity*.

Some patients record long monologues on tape or dictate copious reports to a shorthand writer. A patient of Waxman and Geschwind (1974) imparted his subjective impressions of his illness to a stenographer for a period of 17 hours. The result was a meticulous and lengthy account. Such recordings and dictations are spoken equivalents of the detailed diaries and circumstantial reports of hypergraphics.

Unbridled verbal output

In patients with frontal lobe epilepsy a syndrome of disinhibition, lack of concern, and volatility is sometimes observed. This may be accompanied by periodic aggressive, repetitive or inappropriate verbal behaviour.

Children with acquired verbal pathology and epilepsy

In a number of children, language at first develops normally. Psychomotor development is equally inconspicuous. Then linguistic abilities start to regress. The first symptom is generally a verbal comprehension impairment which may be mistaken for incipient deafness or for an attention disorder. Soon after, expressive disturbances set in. Some children misarticulate or distort words. Others make paraphasias and grammatical errors. Sometimes they use neologisms. Their verbal output may resemble jargonaphasia.

In still other cases, speech production becomes sparse, simplified or telegraphic. At times, verbal output is reduced to a stereotypy: the child produces the same word or syllable whatever (s)he wants to say. For instance, several months after the beginning of the illness, a 4–year-old girl followed up by van Dongen et al. (1977) could utter only the double syllable /tyt-tyt/ when she attempted to communicate verbally.

There are also children who eventually lose all their linguistic abilities. They become globally aphasic. They have to express themselves by means of gestures.

In rare cases, phonology and syntax are relatively preserved but there is a marked impairment of pragmatics: the child's language is linguistically correct but contextually inappropriate – the verbal utterances do not fit the speech situation.

Occasionally, as in a case reported by Nagafuchi et al. (1993), only speech comprehension becomes (severely) impaired, while other linguistic skills, including reading, remain unaffected. The patients have pure (or selective) verbal auditory agnosia.

The acquired deficit sometimes resembles stuttering. In a 7-year-old boy, Deonna et al. (1987) observed slow, protracted and monotonous delivery with hesitations and some iterations. The rest of the boy's linguistic behaviour was completely normal.

The symptomatology, then, is far from being uniform. The disorder may affect all linguistic abilities or only some of them. The impairment may resemble classical motor aphasia (i.e. motor aphasia as it may be observed in adults following brain damage) or classical sensory aphasia or classical global aphasia. It may also mimic aphasia with recurrent utterance. At other times, it is reminiscent of dysarthria, speech apraxia or stuttering.

In addition to inter-individual differences, there may be intra-individual differences, i.e. the type of aphasia may change during the illness. The verbal disorder sometimes undergoes a so-called *Syndromwandel*, a change in symptomatology.

The verbal disability usually begins between 3 and 8 years of age. It is occasionally concomitant with intellectual deterioration or with a mild form of apraxia, i.e. a disturbance of the ability to perform skilled actions. Not infrequently, the difficulty in interpreting verbal stimuli extends after a while to non-verbal sounds, i.e. auditory agnosia develops: in addition to his speech comprehension problem the child loses the ability to identify familiar noises such as a doorbell ringing or a dog barking.

In some children, complete or near complete recovery is observed after some time. In others, recovery – particularly from aphasia – takes years and may remain incomplete; in addition, temporary improvements are not infrequently followed by relapses. In adulthood, sequelae of the aphasia are still noticeable. On the whole, prognosis is poorer when the affliction starts in early childhood. In some cases, the verbal impairment remains so important that sign language has to be used as a substitute for speech (Baynes et al. 1998).

Epileptic seizures set in before or after the beginning of language and/or speech decay. They may consist of partial motor attacks, atypical absences and/or tonic-clonic fits, and their frequency is quite variable. In a minority of cases, epilepsy remains subclinical

The waking EEG findings are diverse: bilateral temporal or temporo-parietal spikes, bilateral slow wave activity over the temporal regions, generalized spike and/or (sharp) slow wave discharges, or multifocal or unilateral spikes. The background rhythm is normal. The epileptic focus is not stable, even though it statistically tends to be in the temporal lobes.

On the other hand, at night a pattern of sustained spikes and waves is commonly observed. As a rule, it does not exceed 85 per cent of total sleeping time.

Since no structural brain lesion can be discovered, the epilepsy is considered cryptogenic (see p. 2).

Seizures and EEG anomalies tend to regress spontaneously until they completely disappear in adolescence. Nonetheless, various treatments are applied in order to reduce the number and severity of seizures as soon as possible. Phenobarbital, carbamazepine and phenytoin have proved ineffective or even aggravating. Valproic acid, ethosuximide and benzodiazepines are moderately effective. The best results have been obtained with corticosteroids (Marescaux et al. 1990). This medication appears particularly effective if it is used during the acute phase of language regression (Tuchman 1994; Tsuru at al. 2000). Intravenous injection of immunoglobin has also been used with some success (Mikati and Saab 2000).

At times, surgery is resorted to: part of the temporal lobe on one side is removed (temporal lobectomy) or the subpial intracortical fibres are transected in one of the temporal lobes (see p. 93).

In the majority of cases, no simple relationship is observed between the seizures and the linguistic deficits. The former may very well diminish or even disappear (spontaneously or under the influence of therapy) while the latter remain.

The condition is encountered more frequently in boys than in girls. Its pathogenesis is still poorly understood. The verbal impairment, the epileptic seizures and the paroxysmal EEG anomalies may all be due to an underlying disturbance of the central nervous system.

When the disorder affects verbal competence, i.e. when it is aphasic in nature, it is usually called *acquired epileptic aphasia* or *acquired aphasia with convulsive disorder*. The condition was described for the first time in 1957 by William Landau and Frank Kleffner. It is therefore often referred to as the *Landau-Kleffner syndrome (LKS)*. This eponym is at times used to denote the whole syndrome of acquired verbal pathology with epilepsy.

Children suffering from the Landau-Kleffner syndrome are sometimes hyperactive, aggressive or depressive. It is not clear whether these behavioural disorders are reactive, i.e. consequent upon the communicative difficulties, or, conversely, due directly to the brain pathology that is also responsible for the verbal impairment and the epilepsy.

There exists another condition that somewhat resembles the Landau-Kleffner syndrome. It features epilepsy concomitant with persistent deterioration of intelligence, memory, attention, temporo-spatial orientation, visuo-spatial abilities and emotional adjustment. The cognitive disintegration is reminiscent of the *Lennox-Gastaut syndrome* (see p. 4). In approximately 50 per cent of the cases, there is in addition an acquired language deficit, the severity of which may be fluctuating. Generalized spike and wave activity can be recorded during over 85 per cent of slow sleep. The condition is therefore called *continuous spikes and waves during (slow) sleep (CSWS) syndrome*.

The CSWS syndrome begins before the age of 10 with a peak around 4 to 5 years old. Until the age of 15, patients have frequent motor seizures.

Corticoids tend to stop them and to normalize nocturnal EEGs. Sometimes, they have a beneficial influence on cognition. However, in many cases, the mental deficit persists preventing the patients from leading a normal life in adulthood.

It is still a matter of dispute whether the Landau-Kleffner syndrome and the syndrome of continuous spikes and waves during slow sleep should be considered two different disorders or two variants of the same illness.

Yet another epileptic syndrome is occasionally associated with acquired speech problems, oral apraxia (which is a difficulty moving part of the mouth or throat on request) and/or writing difficulties. This third syndrome is called *benign partial epilepsy with Rolandic spikes*. It is characterized by infrequent partial motor seizures which occur mainly during sleep. These are not severe and disappear before adolescence. They are therefore considered benign. The EEG in waking state shows focal and multifocal sharp waves in the centro-temporal (Rolandic) regions. These anomalies increase during sleep without, however, exceeding 85 per cent of slow sleep time.

Conclusions

It appears, then, that epilepsy may cause, or be accompanied by, a number of chronic language and/or speech deficits. None of these is uniquely connected with epilepsy, though. Each of them may be encountered in brain-damaged individuals without epilepsy.

Linguistic oddities such as are observed in a number of patients with epilepsy are not specific either. They, too, occur at times in people without epilepsy. Hypergraphia, for instance, is found in a number of non-epileptic mental retardates.

Moreover, there are patients with epilepsy who do not evidence any inter-ictal linguistic disorders or deviations. Indeed, some patients are verbally agile, while others write valuable literary works or memorable epistles (see Chapter 7).

Accordingly, it is not possible to draw a picture of the typical inter-ictal verbal behaviour of patients with epilepsy. Actually, there exists no such characteristic behaviour. No patient can be identified as suffering from epilepsy on the sole basis of their verbal performance or competence.

Epilepsy and literary production

Two nineteenth-century novelists, born in the very same year and dying one year apart from each other, each suffered from epilepsy – and their disorder had a significant influence on their literary production. One was Russian, the other French: they were Fyodor Mikhailovich Dostoevsky and Gustave Flaubert.

Dostoevsky

Dostoevsky's life

Fyodor Mikhailovich Dosto(y)evsky (Figure 7.1) was born in 1821 in Moscow, the son of a surgeon. In childhood, he probably suffered from rickets and scrofula. As a young man, Dostoevsky was relatively short of stature, but had broad shoulders and large hands and feet. He had blond hair, a high forehead and small grey eyes. He became a military engineer, but after a short while he left the army and turned to literature, publishing his first novel, *Poor People*, in 1846.

Dostoevsky joined revolutionary circles in St Petersburg and eventually was arrested. In 1849, he was sentenced to death, but was reprieved at the last moment and sent to hard labour in Siberia. He spent several years in a camp at Omsk in the southern part of Siberia, and then was sent as a soldier to Semipalatinsk in East Kasakhstan. While there, he married a widow, Marya Dmitrevna Isaeva.

In 1859, Dostoevsky returned to St Petersburg and resumed his literary career, producing some of the greatest novels in Russian literature. However, he was plagued with domestic trials and gambling debts. His wife died in 1864, and Dostoevsky married again three years later. Between 1867 and 1871, he and his second wife, Anna Grigorievna, lived in Western Europe. He then returned to St Petersburg where he died of a lung infection in 1881, aged 60.

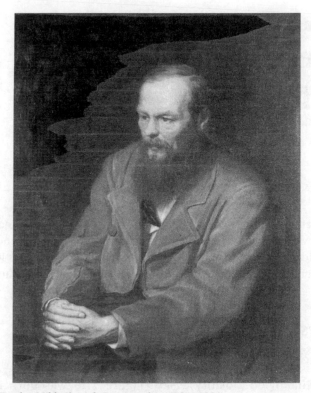

Figure 7.1: Fyodor Mikhailovich Dostoevsky (1821–1881).

Dostoevsky's epilepsy

It is uncertain when precisely Dostoevsky began suffering from epilepsy. It is sometimes assumed that the illness started in childhood, maybe around the age of 7. Initially the seizures seem to have been partial and their epileptic nature, therefore, was not recognized (see pp. 6 and 19). Apparently it was not until 1846 that Dostoevsky had his first generalized convulsive attack in the presence of a witness, his friend Grigorovitch. Between 1847 and 1849 his physician Janowsky witnessed three seizures. A diagnosis of epilepsy could then be made, but it would seem that Dostoevsky heard (or accepted) this diagnosis only later on, when he was in Siberia.

As an adult, Dostoevsky presented with psychomotor spells, which often evolved into secondary generalized convulsions. He also had primary grand mal attacks. Not infrequently he let out a loud cry at the beginning of the access. This cry used to frighten those who heard it for the first time. During the fit there often was froth around Dostoevsky's mouth. Most of these seizures were nocturnal, occurring some time after the writer had fallen asleep. Diurnal attacks with a fall to the ground at times entailed injuries. Post-ictally there could be mental confusion with automatisms. Some seizures were followed by speaking and writing difficulties and memory lapses. There could also be a depressed mood for several days.

The frequency of the accesses varied greatly during Dostoevsky's life. On the whole, they were more frequent after his return from Siberia. However, he seems to have been seizure-free during the last four years of his life. According to his second wife, he was most likely to have attacks when he was vexed or irritated or when he drank alcohol.

Some epileptic fits had an aura. According to two of his acquaintances, Dostoevsky reported that some of his auras were ecstatic: during them he would experience an immense happiness and an intense bliss; he had the impression of a divine touch or revelation. He maintained that Mohammed, who reportedly also suffered from epilepsy, had similar ecstatic auras, during which he felt as if he were in paradise. According to his friends, Dostoevsky claimed that he would not have exchanged his intense ictal felicity for all the joys of the world. Nevertheless, he found his attacks a serious handicap because they interfered with his work and, in his view, could eventually cause apoplexy. The negative aftermath of the seizures increased as he grew older.

In his notebooks and diaries Dostoevsky frequently referred to his epilepsy, particularly after 1860. His biographer J. Frank (1995: 410) has quoted the following passages from the notebook for 1870:

> Crisis at six o'clock in the morning . . . I was not aware of it, woke at eight o'clock with the feeling of an attack. My head ached, my body felt shattered. NB in general the result of an attack, that is, nervousness, weakening of the memory, a state of cloudiness, and some sort of pensiveness – now lasts longer than in previous years. Earlier, this passed in three days, now not before six. In the evening especially, by candlelight, a sick sadness without cause and as if a red coloration, bloody (not a tint) on everything. Almost impossible to work these days . . . An attack while sleeping this morning. I had just fallen asleep [Dostoevsky used to work at night and to sleep through most of the morning]. Anya [his second wife] told me about it at 1.30 . . . My body is not too shattered, but my head even now is still not clear, especially toward evening. Anguish. I remark in general that the attacks even of a moderate kind at present (that is, as I get older) have a greater effect on my head, my brain, than strong attacks in the past.

One of Dostoevsky's children was also afflicted with epilepsy. This child, a boy called Alyosha (Alexis), died during an episode of status epilepticus at the age of 3.

Interpretations of Dostoevsky's epilepsy

Through the years Dostoevsky's epilepsy has been variously construed. Using biographical and autobiographical reports as well as passages from his novels, different researchers have upheld different views of the writer's affliction.

Freud (1927) claimed that Dostoevsky's seizures were actually hysterical fits. Indeed, he considered hysteria the main source of Dostoevsky's literary genius. Hysteria itself had its origin in the writer's psychic constitution as well as in a severe punishment that his father gave him when he was a child, probably because of masturbation. The castigation increased his Oedipus complex. Trying to repress his desire to see his father die, Dostoevsky developed pseudo-seizures as a form of self-punishment.

Freud's psychoanalytical interpretation of Dostoevsky's epilepsy has been criticized by many including Geschwind (1984). Gastaut (1978) called it a 'monstrous error' and Frank (1976) has shown that it is based on incomplete or unreliable reports.

It is nowadays generally agreed that Dostoevsky's illness was true epilepsy. But what kind of epilepsy? Gastaut (1979) upheld the view that the novelist suffered from idiopathic or essential grand mal: his seizures were all primary generalized convulsive attacks. However, they could be ushered in by an absence of the petit mal type or by violent bilateral jerks.

Gastaut further contended that Dostoevsky never had ecstatic auras. Indeed, according to the French epileptologist, auras are never exhilarating, let alone enrapturing. The feeling of elation sometimes experienced by Dostoevsky before he lost consciousness was nothing but an impression of detachment and aloofness caused by the absence.

However, sporadic reports of psychic seizures characterized by a pervading feeling of utter bliss are to be found in the neurological literature (e.g. Alajouanine 1963; Boudouresque et al. 1972; Cirignotta et al. 1980; Landsborough 1987). It could therefore be that, at times, Dostoevsky just prior to losing consciousness really felt, as he himself is reported to have stated, 'in perfect harmony with myself and with the entire universe'. He had the impression 'that the sky had descended to the ground and had swallowed [him] up'.

Admittedly, an ecstatic aura or seizure can never be ascertained objectively. One has to take the patient's word for it. There seems to be no reason, though, to reject the subjective reports of patients who claim that they at times experience a feeling of extreme felicity in the course of an attack.

In addition, there is evidence that Dostoevsky, as he himself indicated in a letter to his brother Michael, had various kinds of epileptic accesses. Beside primary generalized fits, he had psychic and psychomotor episodes, often with secondary generalization. A number of neurologists, including Alajouanine (1963) are of the opinion that Dostoevsky's psychic and psychomotor seizures were manifestations of temporal lobe epilepsy.

Geschwind (1984) pointed out that Dostoevsky was very much concerned with philosophical and religious issues. In addition, the novelist often stressed the importance of morality, even though he himself was far from being a paragon of virtue. Indeed, he was an inveterate gambler. Furthermore, he was irascible and had a low frustration level. He also seems to have had a lack of sense of humour. He was hypergraphic, keeping extensive notebooks and diaries replete with minute or trivial details accompanied by drawings and sketches that were often repetitive. A number of neurologists are of the opinion that such traits of character are frequently encountered in people suffering from temporal lobe epilepsy (see p. 68).

According to his second wife, Dostoevsky insisted on order, particularly on his desk. Excessive orderliness is also regarded by some as a frequent inter-ictal feature of temporal lobe epilepsy.

Finally, his conversion from atheism to Christianity may possibly be related to his temporal lobe epilepsy, as patients with this type of epilepsy are said to be prone to (rapid) conversion (see p. 17)

Epilepsy in Dostoevsky's works

Epilepsy is mentioned in several of Dostoevsky's novels. Some of his characters suffer from the disorder, and their symptoms are described, at times in great detail.

Auras

Prince Myshkin, the hero of the novel entitled *The Idiot*, has ecstatic auras very similar to those Dostoevsky is said to have had. Indeed, the words used by Dostoevsky to depict his beatific experiences to friends of his are very close to those which Myshkin utters in the novel when describing the bliss he sometimes feels at the beginning of an attack.

Kirillov, one of the characters in *The Demons*, reports that at times he feels a brief but intense joy and is able to apprehend the harmony of the universe. His speech partner warns him that this may very well be a form of unsuspected epilepsy.

Not all auras are pleasurable, though. More often than not, those of Dostoevsky's characters who suffer from epilepsy experience fear or have a strange feeling of dejection during seizures. This corresponds to what can be clinically observed: patients report unpleasant ictal moods more frequently than enjoyable ones.

During some of his auras, Myshkin has a modified apperception of time, just as a number of patients report they have during some of theirs.

Psycho-sensory delusions and hallucinations

At one point in *The Idiot*, Myshkin mentions a period in his life during which he had many attacks. He did not feel well between accesses. He remained in a state of constant anxiety. In addition, he had memory disorders as well as an enduring impression of *jamais-vu*: things looked strange to him. 'Everything around me was foreign,' he recalls. Jamais-vu delusions are not infrequently reported by patients who have psychic seizures.

In *The Double*, Dostoevsky describes the upset of a character, Golyadkin, who sees a human figure not far from him and gradually realizes that this figure looks exactly like him. Indeed, the figure is him: Golyadkin is looking at his double, he has a doppelgänger. A similar experience is occasionally reported by people with epilepsy: they have the impression of seeing and sometimes of hearing a person who looks exactly like themselves.

This type of hallucination is called *autoscopy*, *autoscopia* (or *heautoscopia*) or, in French, *vision spéculaire* (mirror vision). Autoscopy consists of the illusory perception of one's own body projected into extracorporeal space. The double may at the same time look identical to, and yet in some respects different from, the patient. On its first occurrence(s), the vision generally causes stupefaction and anguish in the sufferer. It may take place in auras as well as in so-called *équivalents épileptiques*, i.e. ictal psychic states not accompanied by symptoms that an observer can perceive (see p. 5).

At times, patients realize that their doppelgänger is but a chimera, i.e. that they are having a hallucination caused by the illness. In Dostoevsky's novel *The Brothers Karamazov*, one of the characters shouts at his double: 'You're a liar, you're my illness, you're a ghost. Only I don't know how to get rid of you, so I can see that I'll have to put up with you for a while. You're a hallucination.'

Psychomotor seizures

Some of Dostoevsky's characters, particularly in *The Demons*, experience dreamy states or cloudings of consciousness during which they behave incongruously or ragingly. For instance, at a party, Nikolai Vsevolodovich passionately kisses a lady on the lips. At another party, Stavrogin catches one of the guests firmly by the nose and pulls him to the centre of the room. One day without any reason Nikolai bites the ear of an acquaintance. On another occasion he presents with what is now called *raptus epilepticus* (see p. 5) during which be severely cuts himself.

Generalized convulsive seizures

Dostoevsky depicted not only partial attacks but also generalized convulsive seizures. In *The Brothers Karamazov* one may read:

> She did not see him fall, but she heard the shriek – that special shriek, strange, but already familiar to her – the shriek of an epileptic having a seizure . . . They found him at the bottom of the cellar steps, foaming at the mouth, and his body twisting

and thrashing about in convulsions . . . The patient, however, did not come round: the fit ceased for a while, but then recommenced.

In some cases the seizure is unusually long, lasting for several days. 'Once I had an attack that lasted for about three days,' Smerdyakov reports in the same novel. 'The shaking stopped and then started again, and for three whole days I didn't come round.' Smerdyakov thus had status epilepticus, as Dostoevsky is said to have had at least once, and as his little son Alyosha had and apparently died of.

At the beginning of the tonic phase of a generalized convulsive seizure patients not infrequently let out a scream, the so-called *initial epileptic cry* (see p. 4). This shout may sound very strange and may frighten those who hear it for the first time. In *The Idiot*, Dostoevsky says of the cry that it is:

a terrible, quite incredible scream, which is unlike anything else . . . in that scream everything human seems suddenly obliterated, and it is quite impossible, at least very difficult, for an observer to imagine and to admit that it is the man [the patient] himself who is screaming. One gets the impression that it is someone inside the man who is screaming. This, at any rate, is how many people describe their impression.

The last sentence in this quotation shows that Dostoevsky had no first-hand knowledge of how the initial epileptic cry actually sounds like: he knew only what other people had told him about it. As a matter of fact, patients who let out a shriek at the beginning of a convulsive access are usually unaware of it and do not remember it afterwards. Presumably consciousness is already lost at the moment the cry is produced.

However, in *The Idiot*, Dostoevsky describes a generalized seizure at the beginning of which the patient, Myshkin, lets out a cry just before he loses consciousness; afterwards he can remember having shouted involuntarily:

Then suddenly some gulf seemed to open up before him: a blinding inner light flooded his soul. The moment lasted perhaps half a second, yet he clearly and consciously remembered the beginning, the first sound of the dreadful scream, which burst from his chest of its own accord and which he could have done nothing to suppress. Then his consciousness was instantly extinguished and complete darkness set in.

In contrast to most patients, then, Myshkin heard the yell he let out, or at least the beginning of it, and he could remember it afterwards. It could therefore be that his 'dreadful scream' was not an initial epileptic cry but rather a vocalization as is sometimes observed in patients with attacks of frontal lobe origin (see p. 37). As frontal lobe seizures not infrequently evolve into generalized seizures with loss of consciousness (Laskowitz et al. 1995), Myshkin's access may have been a partial attack originating in the frontal lobe but generalizing very quickly.

Post-ictal symptoms

Dostoevsky also described post-ictal symptoms. For instance, in *The Gambler*, he mentioned language and memory disorders as well as dullness of the mind consequent upon a generalized seizure:

> He suffered something in the nature of a fit. He fell unconscious, and afterwards for a week he was almost like a lunatic, babbling incoherent nonsense the whole time . . . He was by now completely incapable of reasoning or even of conducting any kind of serious conversation; if there was any, he got himself out of the difficulty by saying 'Hm!' at every word and nodding his head . . . He had grown very forgetful; he was shockingly absent-minded and had acquired the habit of talking to himself.

In addition, the character developed a tendency to palilalia (see p. 38): 'He would hit on some word or phrase that pleased him and repeat it a hundred of times a day, although it did not correspond at all with either his feelings or his ideas.'

Dostoevsky and epilepsy

Dostoevsky, then, described a wide variety of epileptic symptoms in his oeuvre: different sorts of seizures and of auras as well as diverse ictal behaviours and post-ictal deficits. It may therefore be wondered where his information about epilepsy came from. It is conceivable that part of it was found in medical books. As a matter of fact, Dostoevsky is known to have consulted a number of medical treatises, some of which may have been lent to him by the physicians with whom he was friends. However, most of his information must have been first-hand: he knew about epilepsy because he was afflicted with it. Actually, Dostoevsky described a number of psychomotor, sensory and psychic seizures at a time when the epileptic nature of such seizures had not yet been fully recognized (see p. 19). The hallucinations, peculiar moods and strange behaviours of some of his characters were most probably inspired by his own sensations, feelings and deportments during partial seizures. His epileptic characters' pangs and delusions were his own.

In fact, Dostoevsky seems to have stored up in his memory the various sentiments and states of mind he went through during his psychic accesses. In *The Brothers Karamazov*, he says of an epileptic character:

> Standing there in utter solitude, he seemed lost in thought, but in reality he is not thinking at all but merely 'contemplating'. If you were to nudge him, he would

start and look at you as if he had just woken up, oblivious of his surroundings. True, he would soon snap out of his reverie, but if you were to ask him what he had been thinking about as he stood there, he would probably remember nothing, although that would not stop him from locking away, deep inside him, a memory of the sensations that he had experienced during his contemplation. Those sensations are dear to him, and he probably stores them away instinctively and without conscious thought – why and for what purpose, of course, he does not know: perhaps, after many years of hoarding them, he might unexpectedly throw up everything and go off to Jerusalem as a wandering pilgrim, or perhaps he might suddenly set fire to his native village, or perhaps both.

Although Dostoevsky neither set fire to his birthplace nor wandered to Palestine (though he did spend several years travelling in Europe), he did however preserve memories of his ictal experiences and incorporated them into the texture of his books.

What prompted Dostoevsky to depict epileptic symptoms so frequently? One can think of several reasons why he did so. Maybe by describing the disorder with which he was afflicted he was seeking to somewhat alleviate its negative consequences, particularly the despondency it caused. By projecting his illness into some of his characters, he may have tried to objectify it and thus constrain it or make it more endurable. Indeed, by portraying ecstatic auras he may have attempted to convince himself and others that epilepsy could have a positive side and that persons with epilepsy could apprehend divine mysteries which healthy people were unable to approach. In this sense, epilepsy was truly a 'sacred disease' (see p. 13). Furthermore, in *The Idiot*, Dostoevsky may have wanted to show that contrary to what some of his contemporaries, and notably Cesare Lombroso, maintained, epilepsy was not a taint, let alone a vice. Myshkin, the hero of the novel, is a generous and idealistic man, and yet he suffers from epilepsy.

In a paper published in 1864 in *Epocha*, a journal he was editing with his brother Michael, Dostoevsky argued that epilepsy should not be a cause of infamy (see p. 16). He added that the disease did not prevent one from leading an active life and he pointed out that a number of patients were men of achievement. Dostoevsky himself is proof of this. Even though it interfered more often than not with his daily work as a writer, epilepsy did not prevent him from producing a large number of novels and short stories which won him worldwide fame.

It may even be wondered whether his oeuvre would have been quite the same had he not suffered from epilepsy. Some experts, including Alajouanine (1963), are of the opinion that his experiences as one afflicted with the falling sickness helped shape his *weltanschauung* and thus contributed to the originality and depth of his lifework. This of course does not mean that epilepsy was the source of Dostoevsky's genius. Epilepsy is compatible with genius but it does not create it. The ancient view that epilepsy and artistic talent are closely related (see p. 17) has never been substantiated. Dostoevsky became one of the leading exponents of Russian literature despite his malady, not because of it.

Flaubert

Flaubert's life

Like Dostoevsky, Gustave Flaubert (Figure 7.2) was born in 1821, and like the Russian novelist, he was the son of a surgeon. His family lived in Rouen, Normandy.

As a child, Flaubert had some difficulty learning to read, yet as a teenager he already thought of becoming a writer. To please his family, he went to Paris to study law but after some time gave up his study and turned to writing. From 1846 to 1855 he had a liaison with the poetess and novelist Louise Colet. He soon retired to Croisset, a small place near Rouen, where he wrote most of his works.

His first novel, *Madame Bovary*, appeared in instalments in 1856 in the *Revue de Paris* of which his friend Maxime du Camp was director. The work was considered immoral and its author was prosecuted, only narrowly escaping conviction.

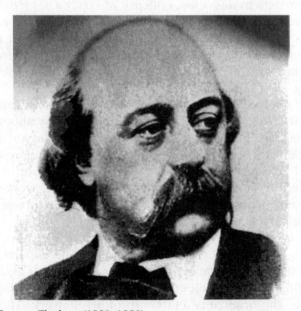

Figure 7.2: Gustave Flaubert (1821–1880).

In his last years, he financially supported his beloved niece Caroline and her husband Ernest Commanville, and his generosity brought him money troubles. He died of a cerebral haemorrhage in 1880, one year before Dostoevsky.

Flaubert did not believe in inspiration. He considered that literary creation was always the result of hard, meticulous and continuous work. He wrote numerous drafts of his novels and these drafts contained lots of corrections. Flaubert was therefore a voluminous writer even though he did not produce a large number of books.

On the other hand, he carried on an extensive correspondence with his mistress Louise Colet, his friend Maxime du Camp and such literati as Guy de Maupassant, George Sand and Théophile Gautier. His edited letters comprise more than ten volumes, despite the fact that most of the numerous letters he wrote to Maxime du Camp were destroyed.

Flaubert's epilepsy

It would seem that Flaubert's epilepsy started when he was a law student in Paris. The seizures were nocturnal and therefore passed unnoticed. The first authenticated attack took place in October 1843. Gustave and his brother Achille, who was a physician like his father, were travelling at night along a small country road near Rouen, in a gig which Gustave was driving. Suddenly, as they were passing another horse-drawn cart and approaching an inn, Gustave had an attack and fell off the gig. He lost consciousness and his brother for a while thought that he was dead. This seizure was followed by a period of frequent epileptic fits. The attacks then became less frequent but apparently never ceased completely.

According to his friend du Camp (1882), Flaubert's diurnal accesses often had an aura with visual phosphenes and anguish: Flaubert would see golden flames or sparks and feel afraid. He was aware of what was happening but was at times unable to speak. Then he would let out a cry, lose consciousness and begin convulsing. After the attack the writer was comatose for a while. There followed a prolonged and deep sleep. When he finally awoke, he used to feel sore all over and this lasted for several days.

In addition to generalized convulsive accesses, Flaubert had psychic seizures during which he would sometimes experience forced thinking or, on the other hand, an avalanche of ideas. At the time, attacks of this type were called 'convulsions of thought' or 'intellectual grand mal'.

There could also be hallucinations. These would usually be accompanied by a feeling of terror and of impending death. At times, the novelist relived the circumstances just prior to his first authenticated fit: he could see himself holding the reins, passing the other cab and watching the light of a distant inn. Not infrequently there was secondary generalization. In addition to these diurnal seizures, Flaubert, like Dostoevsky, had nightly accesses.

According to du Camp, Flaubert avoided referring to his condition as 'epilepsy': he used to speak of his 'nervous attacks'. Flaubert's brother Achille, the physician, considered that the writer suffered mainly from 'épilepsie larvée' (see p. 5).

Epilepsy deeply affected Flaubert's morale and caused him to lead a secluded life at Croisset. Moreover, it slowed down his work as a writer. He tried to compensate for his laborious writing by working long hours, and like Dostoevsky he would often work deep into the night.

Interpretations of Flaubert's epilepsy

Freud construed Dostoevsky's seizures as hysterical fits. René Dumesnil (1905, 1947) and later Jean-Paul Sartre (1971) similarly regarded Flaubert's attacks as pseudo-seizures. However, this interpretation, like Freud's, has been rejected by most experts, who believe that Flaubert was truly epileptic.

Because he had visual auras usually followed by psychic seizures or generalized convulsions, the Gastauts (1982) have argued that Flaubert had an epileptogenic focus in the occipital lobe. Attacks would begin there bringing on phosphenes. Then the abnormal bioelectrical activity would spread to the temporal lobe causing psychic accesses. If the spreading continued, a generalized fit would ensue. As Flaubert evidenced ictal aphasia, the focus must have been in the left hemisphere. The origin of the focus is bound to remain highly conjectural, but if the Gastauts are right and if Flaubert actually had an occipital focus on the left, this focus, or the lesion which caused it, may have been responsible for the trouble the novelist had as a child to learn to read.

In letters to Louise Colet or to friends, Flaubert often complained about a difficulty finding the proper words or constructing adequate sentences. Bart, in his biography of Gustave Flaubert (1967), and the Gastauts (1982) commented that the difficulty may very well have been due to involvement of the left temporal lobe (compare above p. 65).

The temporal involvement may also have been responsible for Flaubert's progressive hyposexuality. While as a young man he had a normal libido, he seems to have gradually become disinterested in sexual activity. Reduced sexuality is often considered an inter-ictal feature of temporal lobe epilepsy. However, as the Gastauts themselves conceded, Flaubert's word-finding difficulties and hyposexuality may also have resulted from the bromide which the writer is said to have regularly taken in order to combat his epilepsy.

Epilepsy in Flaubert's works

In contrast to Dostoevsky, Flaubert made very little use of his illness in his oeuvre. None of his main characters suffers from epilepsy, and there are no detailed descriptions of epileptic seizures in his novels. The only echo of his condition is to be found in the hallucinations that some of his characters, including Emma Bovary, Salammbô, St Anthony, and Frédéric Moreau (in *L'Éducation Sentimentale*), have. These hallucinations are primarily visual and are all, as in Flaubert's case, tinged with anguish. In addition, Emma Bovary has fits or swoons elicited by emotions or smells.

However, in a letter to Louise Colet (quoted in part by the Gastauts, 1982), Flaubert indicated that he was contemplating writing a novel entitled *The Spiral* in which he would detail his experiences as a man afflicted with epilepsy. It is uncertain, though, whether such a book was ever written, or even begun.

Flaubert and epilepsy

As an artist, Gustave Flaubert is generally considered an accomplished stylist, a consummate craftsman, a goldsmith of the written word. Indeed, the form of his novels is often deemed superior to the contents. Would he have produced such finely wrought books if he had not had to struggle with words? Did his painstaking chiselling of sentences and paragraphs not result, at least in part, from the difficulty he experienced finding adequate terms and ordering them to his complete satisfaction? By interfering with the functioning of his brain, particularly of his left temporal lobe, epilepsy, or the bromide he took to combat it, or both combined, may have had a significant impact on his literary production.

On the other hand, it may be wondered whether Flaubert's numerous drafts and very many letters did not to some extent proceed from a nearly irrepressible urge to write. Do they not testify a tendency to hypergraphia, as Dostoevsky's detailed notebooks and diaries seem to do? Maybe Flaubert would not have carried on such an extensive correspondence if he had not suffered from epilepsy.

A similar question can be asked regarding the epistolary activity of another celebrity, Paul the Apostle.

St Paul

St Paul's life

St Paul (Figure 7.3) was born at Tarsus (in the extreme south of present-day Turkey) probably in the first years of the Christian era. His parents were Jews and his first name was Saul. He apparently trained as a rabbi in Jerusalem under Gamaliel, a famous scripturalist. Paul became a fervent Pharisee and a relentless persecutor of the early Christians. He may have attended the stoning to death of St Stephen.

The New Testament (Acts of the Apostles 9: 1–30; 22: 3–21; 26: 12–20) reports that one day, as he was travelling to Damascus with some colleagues, Paul suddenly saw a very bright light and fell to the ground. He then heard

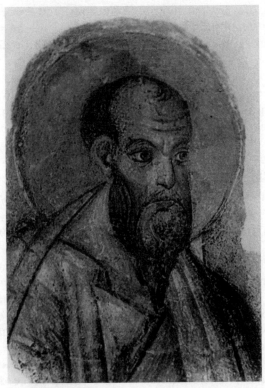

Figure 7.3: St Paul (1st century AD).

(and maybe also saw) Jesus ordering him to serve him instead of persecuting his followers. Paul became immediately blind and had to be led to Damascus by his companions. For three days he could not see, and he did not eat or drink anything. Then a man called Anasias came and by imposing hands on him cured him of his blindness. Paul was then baptized and started to feed himself. He returned to Jerusalem and went to pray in the temple. He fell into a trance and in a vision saw Jesus who ordered him to go and evangelize the Gentiles.

Paul undertook missionary journeys to Cyprus, Asia Minor and Greece. Returning to Jerusalem, he was arrested and imprisoned. As he had Roman citizenship he appealed to Caesar and was transferred to Rome. According to one tradition, he was sentenced to death and executed. Another tradition has it that he was set free and could go to Spain. He probably died between 62 and 65 AD.

Paul is said to have written numerous letters, most of them meant for Christian communities he had visited or helped to create. These letters were generally considered 'weighty and powerful' (2 Corinthians 10: 10). The

New Testament contains 13 so-called Pauline epistles, but most probably they were not all written by Paul.

On the other hand, Paul seems to have had a speech impediment associated with a rather weak physical bearing (2 Corinthians 10: 10), which may have made his public appearances somewhat problematic.

St Paul's epilepsy

Tradition has it that Paul suffered from epilepsy. The condition is therefore sometimes called *galar Phoel*, i.e. 'Paul's illness' in Gaelic (see p. 19). As a matter of fact, the New Testament contains some data which can be interpreted as indicative of epilepsy. In his second epistle to the Corinthians, Paul mentioned that he was plagued with 'a thorn in the flesh', probably a bodily handicap, with which, as he said, the devil racked him. Paul added that he had repeatedly prayed to the Lord that he be relieved of the infirmity, but in vain (12: 7-9). As epilepsy was considered a form of possession (see p. 14), Paul's affliction may very well have been the falling sickness.

In his epistle to the Galatians, the apostle recalled that his brethren had not despised or rejected him on account of his illness, but had received him 'as an angel of God, even as Jesus Christ' (4: 14). Apparently in this passage the words *despised* and *rejected* are the translations of a verb which literally meant 'spat at' (compare Greek *ptuein*, to spit (at), to scorn). The passage, therefore, may be alluding to epilepsy, as people used to spit on epileptics in order to avoid contagion (see p. 16). On the other hand, epileptics were sometimes considered to be prophets directly inspired by God (see p. 17).

In the Acts of the Apostles and in several Pauline letters, visions are mentioned during which Paul saw and/or heard Jesus and received divine revelations. Indeed, in the second epistle to the Corinthians, a man, who turns out to be Paul himself, is said to have experienced an ecstasy which 'caught him up to the third heaven' (12: 2). Such ecstatic visions strikingly resemble Dostoevsky's blissful epileptic auras. It is therefore quite possible that Paul had visual auras or hallucinations of epileptic origin.

On the way to Damascus, Paul's vision may have been followed by a grand mal seizure, since he fell to the ground. And his subsequent blindness may have been post-ictal. Actually, convulsive seizures are occasionally followed by blindness of a few hours' to a few weeks' duration (Landsborough 1987).

Paul may have had another episode of post-ictal blindness during a visit to the Galatians, since in his epistle to them he wrote that 'if it had been possible, you would have plucked out your own eyes, and have given them to me' (4: 15).

Paul was a bachelor who does not seem to have had a strong libido. On the other hand, he had deep religious concerns and his conversion to Christianity seems to have occurred rather suddenly. As was mentioned above, hyposexuality, religiosity and proneness to (quick) conversion are often associated with temporal lobe epilepsy.

Furthermore, the apostle apparently had a quick temper. This trait of character is not infrequent in patients with epilepsy of temporal origin.

Paul is reported to have had a vast epistolary activity. As in Flaubert's case, the extensive correspondence may be viewed as a form of hypergraphia related to epilepsy.

St Paul may very well, therefore, as tradition has it, rank among the famous sufferers from the 'sacred disease'. If he had not been epileptic, he might have written much less and none of his epistles might have survived.

In his first epistle to the Corinthians Paul dealt with glossolalia and claimed that he possessed exceptional ability in the gift of tongues (14: 18). This claim may have reinforced the belief that glossolalia was due to epilepsy. Indeed, Paul may possibly have had seizures during which he involuntarily produced spontaneous neologistic palilalias (see above p. 38) resembling religious glossolalia.

In addition to Flaubert and St Paul, there is yet a third celebrity whose ample correspondence may have been related to epilepsy: Vincent van Gogh.

van Gogh

van Gogh's life

The eldest son of a clergyman, Vincent Willem van Gogh (Figure 7.4) was born in 1853 at Groot-Zundert in the southern part of the Netherlands. As a young man he started to work for an art-dealing company, but soon took a passionate interest in theology and became a lay preacher, first in England and later in the southern part of Belgium. However, his fanaticism made him unpopular. He gave up preaching in 1880 and took to drawing and painting. He returned to his homeland, staying at various places in the Netherlands. He then went to Antwerp, and a little later to Paris where his beloved brother Theo worked as an art dealer. After a while he moved to Arles in Provence where for a few months he lived and worked with another painter, Paul Gauguin. One day, in what looked like a state of frenzy, he attempted to hurt or kill Gauguin. Then he cut off part of his own left ear. Because of this and a series of nervous attacks he was hospitalized, first in Arles and later at Saint-Rémy-de-Provence. After that he moved to Auvers-sur-Oise, near Paris, where he stayed at Dr Gachet's. There he committed suicide in 1890.

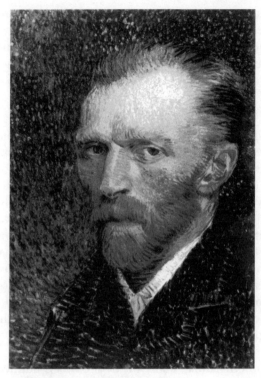

Figure 7.4: Vincent van Gogh (1853–1890).

van Gogh's epilepsy

It is not clear when van Gogh started suffering from epilepsy. Apparently clinical seizures did not begin until 1887. They were psychic, hallucinatory or psychomotor. During psychic attacks the painter would feel horribly anxious or tired and dull. Hallucinations were auditory and/or visual and were often frightening. At times they consisted in the vivid reliving of past events. When they occurred during sleep they were generally experienced as dreadful nightmares.

During psychomotor seizures Vincent would sometimes behave aggressively or shout and gesticulate frantically. It is generally assumed that he assaulted his friend Gauguin and cut his own left ear lobule in the course of a psychomotor access. Complex partial attacks with automatisms could also occur during the night. Van Gogh behaved then like a somnambulist.

Seizures were often followed by temporary confusion. While in this state the painter would sometimes write incomprehensible letters or be agitated and behave erratically. Afterwards, he was generally (partially) amnesic for what he had done during the psychomotor fit and the ensuing confusional state. However, it would seem that van Gogh never had grand mal convulsions. All his attacks were complex partial seizures.

To alleviate his illness, van Gogh was given bromide and warned that alcohol, particularly absinthe (which at the time was much in vogue), had a negative influence on the number and severity of his seizures.

Interpretations of van Gogh's epilepsy

The physicians who examined Vincent van Gogh at the hospital of Arles and at the asylum of Saint-Rémy-de-Provence had no doubt that the painter was suffering from non-convulsive epilepsy. However, this diagnosis was questioned later on and it was proposed that van Gogh had schizophrenia instead. Nowadays it is generally agreed that the artist actually suffered from temporal lobe epilepsy at the end of his short life. This interpretation is based not only on the nature of van Gogh's seizures but also on the observations that he was impulsive and quick-tempered, that as a young man he had deep religious concerns, and that, as he himself reported, he showed hyposexuality during his last years. These features are considered to be often present in people with temporal lobe epilepsy (see p. 68).

As additional evidence, the fact is adduced that van Gogh carried on an extensive correspondence, particularly with his brother Theo. Actually, van Gogh's edited letters encompass three volumes. Moreover, the letters are often long and circumstantial. Many of them contain minute accounts and trivial details. There are also striking word and phrase repetitions. And within a letter, an idea is sometimes expressed several times, or the written text is supplemented with a synonymous sketch. A number of letters are furthermore interspersed with aphorisms. Indeed, van Gogh at times drew up lists of (self-created) apophthegms. All of these features are typical of hypergraphia as it may be observed in a number of patients with temporal lobe epilepsy (see p. 65).

As a painter and drawer too, van Gogh proved extraordinarily productive: between 1880 and 1890 he made over 800 oil paintings and over 700 drawings. Moreover, he often painted or drew the same subject several times (in a row). Few artists have painted as many self-portraits as van Gogh. Quite a number of his canvasses represent a road with a solitary figure. Several times he used a pair of old shoes as his subject, and in the autumn of 1886 and spring of 1887 he repeatedly painted the Moulin de la Galette at Montmartre, Paris. Accordingly, excessive or repetitive epistolary or pictorial activity in people with epilepsy is sometimes called *van Gogh's syndrome*.

Conclusion

It appears then that epilepsy is not incompatible with literary production. Indeed, epilepsy and literary talent may co-exist. The seizures of Dostoevsky and Flaubert may have tended to interfere with their daily work as writers, but did not prevent them from creating masterpieces.

Temporal lobe epilepsy may even induce written overproduction. Epistolary activity may be stimulated by temporal epileptogenic foci. St Paul, Flaubert and van Gogh might not have written so many letters had they not suffered from epilepsy. In fact, if he had not been afflicted with epilepsy, St Paul might never have become one of the main church fathers.

CHAPTER 8

The effect on language of surgery for intractable epilepsy

In a number of patients, epilepsy proves medically refractory, i.e. drugs are unable to noticeably decrease the frequency or the severity of the seizures. This intractable epilepsy may considerably interfere with the patients' education and daily life activities. When this is the case, neurosurgery is sometimes used as a last resort procedure.

If seizures tend to originate from a specific cerebral structure, alleviation of the condition is sometimes attempted by surgical resection of this structure. If the latter is a cortical area, the operation is called *cortectomy* or *topectomy*. If one or several gyri are removed, one speaks of *lobectomy*.

At times, instead of removing part of the cortex, the surgeon cuts the horizontal fibres interconnecting the neurones considered to form the epileptogenic focus. The vertical fibres are spared as are the blood vessels from the pia (which is the innermost membrane investing the brain). This technique, which goes by the name of *(multiple) subpial transection*, is based on the experimental observation that paroxysmal discharges tend to spread along horizontal fibres whereas non-pathological impulses (necessary for the implementation of physiological functions) tend to travel along vertical fibres. The procedure is used primarily when the focus lies in a cortical area whose resection would probably leave the patient with severe motor or linguistic deficits.

If no resectable focus can be identified, or if there are bilateral foci, *callosotomy* is sometimes performed. This operation, which is also called *commissurotomy*, consists in severing the corpus callosum, which is the largest bundle of fibres interconnecting the two cerebral hemispheres. In some cases, the whole bundle is transected. In other cases, only part of the corpus callosum is divided. Complete callosotomy may occur in two stages, part of the callosal fibres being severed during a first operation, and the rest during a subsequent intervention. In some cases, other, less important, fibre tracks interconnecting the two hemispheres (such as the anterior commissure, the massa intermedia, or the hippocampal commissure) are transected

at the same time as the corpus callosum. Patients having undergone callosotomy are often referred to as *split brain patients*.

If epilepsy results from lesions largely confined to one hemisphere and
these lesions also entail motor deficits (such as infantile hemiplegia) and/or
behavioural disorders, *hemispherectomy* is sometimes performed. This
operation consists in removing most of the affected hemisphere, generally
sparing the basal ganglia and possibly some unaffected gyri. If only the cortex
is resected while the underlying white matter is largely preserved, the intervention is called *hemidecortication*.

These various forms of surgery for intractable epilepsy often result in a
reduction of seizure frequency and severity and/or in increased efficacy of
anticonvulsant therapy. However, after callosotomy, focal seizures may
occur which were not observed before surgery. Even if it is followed by
such seizures, the operation is nevertheless considered beneficial if it has
put an end to generalized seizures or has markedly reduced their
frequency.

Cortectomy, lobectomy, multiple subpial transection, callosotomy,
hemispherectomy and hemidecortication may all have transient or durable
effects on language.

Language after cortectomy or lobectomy

When part of the temporal cortex or of the temporal lobe is resected,
patients not infrequently show an impairment of *verbal memory*, i.e. of the
ability to remember lists of words or stories. Usually, the impairment is more
pronounced if the operation has been performed on the left temporal lobe. If
pre-operatively there already was a reduction of verbal memory (see above,
p. 65), an aggravation of the deficit is generally observed after surgery.
However, with the passing of time, the disability may reach its pre-operative
level again, particularly if the patient is seizure-free after operation (Novelly
et al. 1984; Ojemann and Dodrill 1985; Zaidel et al. 1994).

Occasionally, however, verbal memory proves to be better after surgery
than before, but for this to be the case the resection must have been
performed on the right side and the patient must have significantly fewer
seizures than before operation. The most likely explanation for the improvement is that the epileptogenic focus in the right temporal lobe interfered
with the verbal memory functions of the left temporal lobe. Once the focus is
removed, the number of seizures decreases, sometimes to zero, and the
performance of the left temporal lobe is no longer hampered.

Anterior temporal lobectomy on the left may not only impair verbal
memory, but it may also entail lasting *anomia*, i.e. persistent word-finding
difficulties.

Milner et al. (1964) observed severe post-operative aphasia following right temporal lobectomy in a patient with no definite hand preference. There were no comprehension difficulties, but speech and writing were grossly impaired, with neologisms, spelling errors and grammatical mistakes that made the patient's verbal output difficult to understand. The patient, a well-educated man, was aware of his expressive impairment but could not correct himself.

On the other hand, in a few patients with epilepsy and chronic stuttering (see p. 58), it was noted that right temporal lobectomy resulted in normalization of speech delivery (Guillaume et al. 1957; Mazars et al. 1970). And in children with severe acquired epileptic aphasia (see p. 71), partial recovery of linguistic skills is sometimes observed after removal of the anterior part of the temporal lobe (Cole et al. 1988). In children with underdeveloped verbal abilities, temporal lobectomy performed in the few years following the onset of seizures may result in an improvement of the verbal IQ (Meyer et al. 1986).

Following surgery on the frontal lobe, there may be a reduction of *verbal fluency*, i.e. of the ability to generate lists of nouns beginning with a specified letter or belonging to a specified semantic category. Such reduction is more likely to occur after left-sided than after right-sided surgery.

Patients who have undergone frontal lobectomy may also show *verbal aspontaneity*, i.e. a reduction in verbal output and in inclination to engage in verbal intercourse.

In some patients, then, cortectomy and lobectomy, reflect negatively on linguistic or metalinguistic performance. Metalinguistic skills are abilities, such as verbal fluency, which are gauged by verbal tests but do not seem indispensable for the daily use of language in communicative situations. In other cases, on the contrary, surgery results in an improvement of (a number of) verbal skills.

Language after multiple subpial transection

In children with severe acquired epileptic aphasia (see p. 71), total or partial recovery of verbal functions is sometimes observed following transection of horizontal intracortical fibres underlying the epileptogenic focus (Morrell et al. 1995). Nass et al. (1999) noted that, when there is improvement, it is generally more perceptible in speech comprehension than in speech production. Moreover, the improvement may be only transitory.

Language after commissurotomy

Mutism

Following commissurotomy there often is transient mutism. This mutism may last up to one month. In rare cases, it lasts several months. Patients with post-callosotomy mutism understand simple speech and possibly written language but do not speak.

In some cases, mutism is not total: after much urging one occasionally succeeds in eliciting one-word answers from the patient. On the other hand, mutism may be accompanied by akinesia or bradykinesia, that is to say, that the patient moves very little or moves slowly.

Emotional utterances are sometimes observed in mute commissur-otomized subjects. Postoperatively, a split-brain patient of Bogen's (1976) was completely mute. She had no spontaneous speech and could not be made to answer questions or to repeat words. Yet, one day, as an examining physician was urging her to stick out her tongue, she exclaimed: 'Shame on you!'

Recovery from mutism usually goes through a stage of aphonia, during which the patient produces whispered speech. This stage may be followed by a spell of hoarseness, before normal voice production is recovered (Bogen 1976).

The pathogenesis of post-commissurotomy mutism is still poorly under-stood. In particular, it is not clear whether speechlessness results directly from the interruption of interhemispheric communication or instead from damage that surgery has caused to cerebral structures near the corpus callosum. That such extracallosal lesions may occur has been documented with magnetic resonance imaging (e.g. by Risse et al. 1989).

Writing

Mute split-brain patients are often able to answer simple questions in writing. However, their short answers may contain duplications and omissions of strokes, letters, figures, and syllables (Bogen 1976). The writing disorder may outlive the speechlessness.

Left hand anomia (or aphasia)

In many split-brain patients, a more durable deficit has been reported under the name of *left hand anomia* or *left hand aphasia*. Persons with this deficit are unable to name, or they name incorrectly, objects that they are holding in their left hand with vision occluded. They are also unable to describe these objects verbally or else they give inappropriate descriptions. By contrast, naming and verbal description of objects held in the right hand are correct.

Anomia or aphasia of the left hand in split-brain patients is usually explained in the following way: tactile sensations from the left hand reach the right hemisphere, which identifies the object held by the left hand. However, because it cannot output speech, the right hemisphere is unable to name the object or to provide a verbal description of it. Only the left hemisphere, which is dominant for language, can produce names or verbal descriptions. Since it is now disconnected from the right hemisphere, the left hemisphere cannot share the knowledge which the right hemisphere has of the object held by the left hand. Therefore the left hemisphere is unable to name this object and to describe it verbally. All it can do is to guess at the object. Its wild guesses are often wrong and entail incorrect namings or inappropriate verbal descriptions. Anomia or aphasia of the left hand, then, is a *disconnection* phenomenon, i.e. it results from the lack of communication between the two hemispheres. The area in the right hemisphere where the tactile sensations from the left hand are identified is disconnected from the language area in the left hemisphere. Left hand anomia is a *tactile–verbal disconnection syndrome*.

This view does away with the unity of consciousness, since it implies that the right hemisphere can have some information which the left hemisphere does not share. The commissurotomized patient, then, has ceased to be an individual, i.e. an undivided entity. He or she is a split person with two separate cerebral hemispheres, which receive and process information independently of one another.

Left hand apraxia to verbal commands

Another unilateral deficit that is often observed after callosotomy is *left hand apraxia to verbal commands*. Patients with this impairment are unable to execute, or execute incorrectly, orders which are given orally to be carried out with the left hand. In some cases, the apraxia is limited to the left fingers. In contrast to left hand anomia, which tends to be durable, left hand apraxia to verbal commands usually decreases with the passing of time.

Left hand apraxia for verbal orders is generally explained in much the same way as left hand anomia. It is maintained that under normal circumstances the left hemisphere, having decoded the verbal order, passes the necessary motor instructions to the right hemisphere, which then directs the left hand accordingly. In split-brain patients the transfer of instructions from the left to the right hemisphere can no longer be implemented. The right hemisphere is left to its own devices. As it cannot decode the verbal order properly, it misdirects the left hand.

If the apraxia decreases with the passing of time, it is generally assumed that the patient is gradually learning to innervate the left hand directly from the left hemisphere, or that his/her right hemisphere is acquiring verbal comprehension.

However, the disconnection theory of left hand apraxia to verbal commands fails to account for a number of observations. For instance, some patients with left hand apraxia to verbal commands have difficulty performing gestures not only on verbal order but also on imitation. Their left hand movements tend to be inadequate not only when they are told what to do but also when they are shown what to do (Bogen 1976). How is this double difficulty to be explained? What prevents the patients from reproducing the gestures shown by the examiner? Why do they fail in a test that does not involve language?

Also, patients may be unable to reproduce with the left hand gestures which they have just been performing with the right hand (Bogen and Vogel 1975; Bogen 1976), or, when blindfolded, they may have trouble reproducing on the left a particular configuration of their right hand, even though they have been allowed to feel this configuration with their left hand (Bogen 1976). These patients' right hemisphere has seen the gesture made, or has felt the posture assumed, by the right hand. Why then is it unable to have the left hand reproduce this gesture or this posture?

Again, some patients find it difficult to use their left hand efficiently not only when they obey verbal commands, but also when they are requested to pay attention to the performance of their left hand in manual activities. The husband of a commissurotomized woman once remarked that his wife could use her left hand appropriately in daily actions as long as she did not watch what her left hand was doing. However, difficulties arose as soon as she concentrated on her left hand's performance (Bogen 1976). Why could this patient use her left hand routinely but not heedfully?

Since none of these various questions can be answered satisfactorily on the basis of the disconnection theory, one is justified, it would seem, in looking for an alternative explanation. In fact, when commissurotomized patients evidence post-operative neurological deficits, these deficits tend to be more pronounced or more durable on the left than on the right side. For instance, hypotonia is usually more marked in the left than in the right body half (Gazzaniga et al. 1967). The plantar reflex is generally pathological on both sides, but is more so on the left than on the right (Bogen 1976), or it reverts to normal later on the left than on the right (Gazzaniga et al. 1967). A pathological grasping reflex is observed more frequently or more durably in the left than in the right hand (Ross et al. 1984). Transitory hemi- or monoparesis affects the left side of the body more often than the right side (Baynes et al. 1992; Gur et al. 1984; Ross et al. 1984). And there may be left unilateral neglect (Gur et al. 1984; Novelly and Lifrak 1985), while right unilateral neglect has never been reported.

These neurological asymmetries indicate that following commissurotomy, the functioning of the right hemisphere tends to be more impaired than the functioning of the left hemisphere. This is probably due to the fact that during the operation the right hemisphere is generally more exposed than the left, craniotomy impinging more on the right than on the left half of the skull (Marino et al. 1985: see in particular their Figure 3; Gates et al. 1985: see in particular their Figure 3A; Risse et al. 1989). In addition, during surgery the right hemisphere is usually more retracted to the side than the left hemisphere (Akelaitis et al. 1942; Bogen 1976; Gazzaniga et al. 1967; Novelly and Lifrak 1985; Roberts 1985; Ross et al. 1984). Accordingly, the right half of the brain tends to suffer more bruising than the left half in the course of a callosotomy.

The greater post-operative impairment of the right hemisphere is confirmed by the observation that, when there is a writing disorder after commissurotomy, this disorder is similar to the disturbance of writing which is commonly noted in patients having suffered right brain damage (Lebrun 1985; Ellis et al. 1987).

A number of split-brain patients show conversational inappropriateness. They appear self-centred in verbal intercourse, tend to abruptly change topics and are prone to confabulation (Zaidel 1990). Similar features are not infrequently observed in patients with right brain lesions (Lebrun 1983).

Again, commissurotomized patients not infrequently complain of avocalia, i.e. a loss or reduction of their ability to sing (Bogen and Vogel 1975). This complaint too points to a dysfunction of the right hemisphere, as selective avocalia, i.e. avocalia without speech disorder, usually results from damage to the right half of the brain.

Also, in patients with documented pre-operative right hemisphere dysfunction, the deficit is often found to have increased after surgery (Novelly and Lifrak 1985). The performance Wechsler intelligence quotient, considered to primarily reflect right hemisphere activity, is generally diminished post-operatively, whether it was normal or below norm pre-operatively (Campbell et al. 1981; Zaidel 1990). In contrast, the verbal IQ, thought to reflect left hemisphere activity, is either not or only minimally affected by callosotomy, except in right-handed patients with right hemisphere dominance for language as shown by the Wada technique (see below p. 105). In these patients, the verbal IQ, which depends primarily on the right hemisphere, is depressed after transection of the corpus callosum. In addition, the patients present with obvious aphasic symptoms (Sass et al. 1990).

Frequently, then, the right hemisphere is impaired following callosotomy, and this impairment may very well account for the various difficulties thatpatients experience in the efficient use of their left hand. In all likelihood, left hand apraxia or left hand clumsiness such as is observed in a number of commissurotomized patients is due to post-operative dysfunction of the right hemisphere rather than to interhemispheric disconnection.

It may be wondered whether right hemisphere pathology, in addition to being the cause of left hand apraxia, might not also be responsible for left hand anomia. Could it be that the inability to adequately name or describe an object held in the left hand in fact results from incomplete or faulty identification of the object by the right hemisphere?

This question is generally answered in the negative by the proponents of the disconnection theory on the grounds that patients with left hand anomia, after they have palpated an object with the left hand, keeping their eyes closed, are generally able to retrieve this object from an array of objects which they explore with their left hand. It must therefore be assumed that the object has been identified.

To this it can be replied that identification is not an all-or-none phenomenon. There are various degrees in identification. Identification of a stimulus, particularly by a brain-damaged subject, may remain partial or subliminal, i.e. recognition may be incomplete or may take place without the subject becoming (fully) aware of it.

Retrieval of a palpated object from a limited array can be achieved on the basis of a few features such as general shape, weight or texture. It does not require (complete) identification, as a case described by Platz (1996) shows.

Tactile retrieval may also take place on the basis of unconscious identification. Numerous examples of so-called covert or tacit awareness of stimuli are to be found in the neurological literature. In split-brain patients, such subconscious identification or even perception may be present on the left side. For instance, a commissurotomized patient of Gazzaniga et al. (1963), when requested to show with his left hand which part of his left body half had been touched by the examiner, would sometimes move his hand to the touched body part while simultaneously denying having been touched. Another patient occasionally failed to notice that an object had been placed in his left hand (Gazzaniga and Sperry 1967). Again, if two different letters are simultaneously flashed, one in their left and one in their right visual half-field, some split-brain patients recognize the letter tachistoscopically presented in their right visual half-field (which projects to their left hemisphere), while denying having seen anything on the left. If they are nevertheless requested to choose a letter with their left hand from an unseen array of three-dimensional letters, they consistently select the letter that has been flashed in their left visual half-field (which projects to their right hemisphere), thus demonstrating that they have perceived the left-sided stimulus but are not aware of it (Sperry et al. 1969).

Incomplete or subliminal identification, then, may be quite sufficient for tactile retrieval. Naming, on the contrary, appears to require full and conscious recognition of the stimulus.

Exponents of the disconnection theory of left hand anomia also point out that split-brain patients who cannot name adequately an object held in their left hand with vision occluded, at times make a gesture which is reminiscent of the use of the object. In their opinion, this gesture indicates that the object has been recognized. However, truly agnosic patients, i.e. patients with an unquestionable disorder of recognition, may at times hold a utensil appropriately or activate the movable parts of it, even though they cannot achieve conscious identification of the utensil. Man-made objects have an 'affordance' which may easily call forth a roughly appropriate motor response even in the absence of conscious identification. The physical properties of such objects, including their moveable parts, can elicit movements simulating the effective handling of the objects, even if the subject fails to retrieve their exact nature and/or function (Sirigu et al. 1991). Accordingly, when patients supposed to have left hand anomia make a gesture that is somewhat reminiscent of the use of the object they are holding in their left hand, this gesture cannot be safely regarded as evidence that they have fully identified the object.

An observation made by Barbizet et al. (1974) in patients with an ischemic lesion of the corpus callosum is worth mentioning in this context. The authors found that some of these patients, when they have misnamed an object held in their left hand and are then asked to demonstrate the use of the object while still keeping their eyes closed, make movements in accordance with their misnaming. If it is assumed that in these patients identification of the object to be named has taken place adequately, how can one explain that their right hemisphere directs the left hand in accordance with the erroneous verbal response of the left hemisphere rather than in accordance with the tactile information it has received from the left hand and the identification it is supposed to have performed on the basis of this information? The answer to this riddle is probably to be found in the fact that ischemic lesions of the corpus callosum more often than not also affect adjacent hemispheric structures. And if the right hemisphere is partly damaged, it may conceivably find it difficult to identify objects held in the left hand, imperfect identification leading to misnaming. In other words, the injured right hemisphere is affected with tactile agnosia.

Since in split-brain patients the right hemisphere is frequently bruised during an operation (see above), it too may show (some degree of) tactile agnosia, and its recognition deficit may very well be responsible for the so-called anomia or aphasia of the left hand.

The idea that right hemisphere dysfunction is the cause of apraxia and anomia of the left hand receives additional support from an observation made by Risse et al. (1989), who tested seven patients having undergone partial commissurotomy. Only two of these patients were found to have anomia of the left and/or apraxia of the left hand to verbal commands. Interestingly, in the course of operating on these seven patients, moderate retraction of both hemispheres had been applied instead of the usual more forceful retraction of the right hemisphere only. Therefore, in these patients the right hemisphere is likely to have been less bruised than in other operations and this may well account for the absence of post-operative anomia of the left hand and of apraxia of the left hand to verbal commands in five of them. Moreover, in one of the two patients who did evidence these two deficits of the left hand, MRI investigation disclosed some right brain pathology, and this pathology may certainly account for the impairment of the left hand. In the other patient, no sign of right brain pathology could be detected by means of MRI, but this patient had by far the lowest post-operative full scale IQ of the whole group: 55. This low score may have been partly due to a depressed performance IQ, usually considered to be a sign of right brain impairment.

It would seem, then, that if care is taken to spare the right hemisphere as much as possible during surgery, the risk of having anomia of the left hand or apraxia of the left hand to verbal instructions post-operatively is considerably reduced. This confirms the view that in split-brain patients anomia of the left hand and apraxia of the left hand to verbal commands are likely to be due to right hemisphere dysfunction rather than to the callosal transection per se. This amounts to saying that the two deficits are not disconnection symptoms and are not verbal in nature.

Left hand agraphia

Yet another deficit that is often present in split-brain patients is left hand agraphia, an inability to form letters or to spell words correctly with the left hand. This disorder may be observed even in patients who could write easily with their left hand before operation (Bogen 1976). Indeed, it may occur in left-handers who have always used their left hand in writing. Post-operative left hand agraphia may force these patients to become right-handed for writing (Gur et al. 1984).

Left hand agraphia is generally regarded as a disconnection symptom. Because the right hemisphere does not know how to write, it is dependent on the left hemisphere for the required instructions when the subject wants to write with the left hand. After callosotomy, writing instructions can no longer be transferred from the left to the right hemisphere. Accordingly, the left hand can no longer be directed adequately.

However, since so-called left hand anomia and left hand apraxia to verbal commands can be better explained as deficits due to right hemisphere dysfunction than as disconnection symptoms, it may be wondered whether left hand agraphia might not equally result from post-operative impairment of the right half of the brain.

In conclusion, commissurotomy may disturb the efficient use of language in various ways. The verbal disorders usually decrease or clear up with the passing of time. Their patho-physiology is not yet fully understood. They seem to be due to damage suffered by the right cerebral hemisphere during operation rather than to interhemispheric disconnection, as has been generally assumed.

Improvement of linguistic performances after callosotomy in children with the Landau-Kleffner syndrome

Garcia-Flores (1999) performed partial or total callosotomy in 17 children suffering from the Landau-Kleffner syndrome (see above, p. 71). The operation resulted in improved linguistic performances in patients commissurotomized before the age of 8 years. Apparently, the favourable outcome was due to the fact that callosal transection prevented paroxysmal discharges originating in the left temporal lobe from bringing about an epileptogenic focus in the right temporal lobe. The emergence of an epileptogenic focus in originally healthy cerebral tissue under the influence of a distant, possibly contralateral, focus is called *kindling* or *secondary epileptogenesis*.

Language after hemispherectomy or hemidecortication

In individuals with intractable epilepsy originating from one severely damaged hemisphere, the affected hemisphere, or most of it, is sometimes removed. At times, only the cortex is excised, while the underlying white matter is preserved. Either operation may or may not be followed by a change in the patient's verbal competence.

A number of patients considered for hemispherectomy or hemidecortication are mentally retarded and their ability to use language as a means of communication is commensurate with their level of intellectual achievement: i.e. they have underdeveloped verbal skills on a par with their overall mental deficiency. After surgery, limited or no linguistic improvement is observed, although epilepsy is generally improved. Presumably, in these patients the remaining hemisphere is not intact, and therefore significant progress in cognitive functioning is precluded.

Conversely, there are cases where hemispherectomy is followed by the emergence of language (Heuyer and Feld 1954; Vharga-Khadem et al. 1997) or by a significant improvement in verbal skills (McFie 1961). Indeed, these skills may eventually normalize (Damasio et al. 1975). It is hypothesized that in these patients the affected hemisphere and/or the seizures it provoked impeded or slowed down language development in the intact hemisphere. This negative influence was perhaps enhanced by the anticonvulsant therapy. Following removal of the damaged side and gradual withdrawal of anti-epileptic medication, command of language can be achieved.

However, despite dramatic changes observed shortly after surgery, further development of verbal skills seems in such cases to proceed at a slower pace than in subjects with an intact brain. It looks as if an isolated hemisphere needs more time to reach linguistic proficiency (Lebrun and Leleux 1979). Indeed, some metalinguistic abilities may never fully develop, particularly if it is the left hemisphere that has been excised (Dennis and Kohn 1975; Dennis and Whitaker 1976; Ogden 1996; Vargha-Khadem et al. 1997).

In patients without pre-operative linguistic deficits, surgery may yet be followed by a further development of verbal competence. A patient of Griffith and Davidson (1966) started having seizures at the age of 10 and left hemiplegia at 12. A right hemispherectomy was performed when he was 19 years old. Before operation, the patient's verbal IQ was 101. One year after operation it was 119, and some 15 years later 121. In addition, post-operatively the patient was less verbose and less digressive than before surgery.

From time to time hemispherectomees are encountered who stutter (Leleux and Lebrun 1981). The existence of such patients casts serious doubt on the validity of the theory (Orton 1927, 1928; Jones 1966, 1967; Travis 1978) that stuttering is due to rivalry between the two cerebral hemispheres. Since in hemispherectomized or hemidecorticated patients one hemisphere has been removed or made inoperative, dysfluent speech cannot be the result of interhemispheric competition.

On the other hand, the existence of such patients is compatible with the theory that ascribes stuttering to inadequate cortical control over subcortical nuclei (Lebrun 1997a, 1997b). Indeed, by removing half of the pallium while preserving subcortical nuclei, hemispherectomy and hemidecortication may conceivably reduce cortical control over these nuclei and thus facilitate the occurrence of a stutter, as seems to have been the case in the two patients described by Leleux and Lebrun (1981).

Conclusions

Surgery for intractable epilepsy, then, may influence verbal competence and verbal performance in various ways. At times, the operation is followed by an improvement of linguistic functioning. In other cases, surgery entails temporary or more durable verbal deficits.

Post-operative deficits depend, to a large extent, on the type of operation: verbal disorders observed after cortectomy or lobectomy are different from those observed after commissurotomy or hemispherectomy. Following commissurotomy, linguistic sequelae, if present, are nearly always negative. Fortunately, they are often transitory. On the contrary, cortectomy and hemispherectomy may have a positive or a negative impact or no impact at all on verbal behaviour. When present, negative effects may or may not be durable.

The possibility of there being a prolonged verbal handicap following neurosurgical intervention should be taken into consideration when an operation is being considered.

CHAPTER 9

Verbal behaviour during hemispheric anaesthetization and cortical electrostimulation

When, in an attempt to alleviate intractable epilepsy, a neurosurgeon resects part of the brain, he must be cautious not to impinge on areas that are indispensable for the use of language. Encroaching on these areas might cause durable aphasia or chronic impairment of short-term verbal memory. It is therefore mandatory to spare the so-called 'eloquent' portions of the cerebral cortex, lest the cure be worse than the disease.

Essentially, two methods have been developed to minimize the risk of permanently compromising the patient's verbal skills: hemispheric anaesthetization and cortical electrostimulation. Either method is used in conscious patients as it implies their active participation.

Hemispheric anaesthetization

When aphasia results from a cortical lesion, this lesion usually involves the posterior part of the frontal lobe and/or the superior part of the temporal lobe. Moreover, in right-handers it is generally located in the left hemisphere. In the majority of left-handers, it also lies in the left hemisphere. Only a very limited number of right-handers and a minority of left-handers become aphasic following damage to the right hemisphere.

Accordingly, if in a right-handed patient with intractable epilepsy a resectable epileptogenic focus has been found in the posterior part of the left frontal lobe or the superior part of the left temporal lobe, it is highly desirable to anticipate the possible effect of the envisaged neurosurgery on verbal abilities. The same holds true in respect of left-handers or ambidexters (i.e. subjects with no definite hand preference) with a focus in the posterior part of the frontal lobe or the superior part of the temporal lobe whether on the left or on the right side.

The Wada technique

Predicting the possible impact of cortectomy or lobectomy on linguistic performance can be done by temporarily incapacitating the hemisphere considered for operation. Such incapacitation is achieved by injecting a barbiturate (usually sodium amobarbital) into the cervical portion of the common or internal carotid artery on the side to be tested. The barbiturate is carried by the blood to the cerebral hemisphere which, as a result, is temporarily anaesthetized. The anaesthetization interferes with the functioning of the hemisphere. The occurrence of a contralateral hemiplegia testifies to the disablement.

Provided the injection does not induce obnubilation or drowsiness, the patient is then given a few simple verbal tasks such as repeating sentences, naming pictures of familiar objects, producing serial speech or remembering verbal items used a little earlier. If verbal performances are unremarkable, it is concluded that the anaesthetized hemisphere does not play a leading part in the use of language. If, on the contrary, patients evidence language problems such as aphasia, anomia, paraphasia, perseveration, or inability to remember verbal items, it is concluded that the anaesthetized hemisphere plays an important role in linguistic functions. In order to cross-check the results of the test, the procedure is usually repeated on the other side a day or so later.

This technique of hemispheric anaesthetization was introduced in the late 1940s by Juhn Wada, a Japanese-Canadian neurologist. It is therefore often referred to as the *Wada technique*. The method is not completely innocuous, as puncture of the carotid artery is painful and is never fully risk-free. Consequently, in a number of centres, physicians do not puncture the carotid artery but introduce a catheter into the femoral artery and advance it under fluoroscopic guidance to the internal carotid artery. The barbiturate is administered through the catheter.

The Wada technique is not totally foolproof either. Following surgery there may at times be aphasia even though there was none during temporary anaesthetization of the hemisphere. The discrepancy between the test results and the consequences of the neurosurgical resection may in some cases be due to the fact that the use of language in actual communicative situations is more complex than the use of language during the relatively simple verbal tests of the Wada procedure. The discrepancy may also be due to an uneven distribution of the barbiturate in the cerebral territory irrigated by the branches of the internal carotid artery, i.e. the excised area may not have been fully incapacitated at the time of the injection.

Again, when the Wada technique is used there is always the possibility of part of the barbiturate passing to the contralateral hemisphere via the anterior communicating artery. This hazard is called *cross-filling*. If cross-filling takes place, the functions of the contralateral hemisphere may be interfered with. If the patient then shows signs of aphasia, one cannot make out in which of the two brain halves the verbal disorder originates, and the Wada test remains inconclusive.

In order to check for cross-filling, an EEG can be recorded on the side opposite the injection. If the EEG shows clear signs of perturbation during administration of the test, it is concluded that part of the barbiturate has crossed the midline and the examination is considered invalid.

One can also check for cross-flow by performing an angiogram: a contrast or radioactive product is injected into the carotid artery together with the barbiturate and the brain vessels are visualized to determine whether part of the product passes to the other side of the brain.

Hemispheric dominance for language

Comparison of patients having unilateral brain lesions and aphasia with patients having unilateral brain lesions and no aphasia has given rise to the concept of hemispheric dominance for language. This concept implies that in most individuals one of the two cerebral hemispheres plays a leading part in verbal activities, with the other performing but a complementary or ancillary function. The leading hemisphere is said to be dominant for language.

Comparison of right-handed patients having suffered unilateral brain damage with left-handed patients having suffered unilateral brain damage has led to the conclusion that in the vast majority of healthy right-handers the left hemisphere is dominant for language. Only a few right-handers have right hemisphere language dominance (so-called *crossed dominance*). In the majority of left-handers and ambidexters, the left hemisphere is equally dominant for language. However, the number of left-handers and ambidexters with right hemisphere dominance is far from being negligible. Moreover, in left-handers and ambidexters hemispheric dominance seems to be less pronounced than in strongly right-handed people (see above p. 30). Indeed, a number of non-right-handers are considered to have bilateral representation of language: their two cerebral hemispheres are involved in language processing to more or less the same degree.

In right-handers with epilepsy, the Wada test usually reveals a left hemisphere dominance for language. However, the proportion of patients with right hemisphere dominance is higher than in the healthy population. For instance, in a study by Milner et al. (1964), as many as 10 per cent of the right-handed patients had right hemisphere dominance for language.

The majority of left-handers and ambidexters with epilepsy in whom no evidence of early brain damage can be found also prove to have left hemisphere dominance on the Wada test. The reverse is observed in left-handers and ambidexters with evidence of early brain damage. Presumably, the cerebral lesions incurred in infancy have induced a shift of hemispheric dominance to the right in many of them.

A number of patients show aphasic signs following injection on the left as well as following injection on the right side. However, their transitory aphasia is generally less severe than in patients who evidence aphasia after injection on one side but not after injection on the other side. When aphasia is present whichever side is injected, it is concluded that the patient has bilateral language representation. This feature is observed primarily in left-handed patients and in patients with no clear hand preference.

More often than not, a brief episode of muteness is observed immediately following injection of the barbiturate, irrespective of the side being injected. In other words, anaesthetization of even the non-dominant hemisphere may initially prevent the patient from producing speech. This finding can be related to the observation that speech arrests may occur in patients with an epileptogenic focus in either hemisphere (see above, p. 30).

Cortical electrostimulation

If a patient with intractable epilepsy has a demonstrable epileptogenic focus located in the hemisphere that has been found on the Wada test to be non-dominant for language, resection of the focus will generally be performed. If, on the contrary, the focus lies in the hemisphere found to be dominant for language or if the results of the Wada test are inconclusive, the neurosurgeon may either abandon the idea of operating on that hemisphere or perform a conservative excision, i.e. resect as small an area as possible. He/she may also decide to let the excision be guided by the results of cortical electrostimulation.

For cortical electrostimulation, patients are craniotomized under local anaesthesia and various parts of the exposed cortex are successively stimulated by means of a volley of brief electric pulses of low intensity. Ordinarily an intensity of 3 to 8 mAmp with a pulse duration of 1 to 2 msec is used. If the currents interfere with the performance of simple verbal tasks or with the retention of simple verbal material, it is concluded that the stimulated site plays a critical role in linguistic functions and therefore should, as far as possible, be preserved.

Speech arrests

Electrostimulation may cause speech arrests. Patients are rendered mute. Though unable to speak they may yet be able to move their tongue or lips, to write and to follow verbal instructions. A patient of Penfield and Welch (1951) who had had a speech arrest caused by stimulation, said afterwards to the physician: 'I could hear what you were saying, doctor. I knew what I wanted to say, but I just couldn't.'

If stimulation takes place while patients are talking, they stop speaking but can generally proceed with their interrupted utterance upon cessation of the current. If they are counting aloud when stimulation is applied, there is a break in the recitation that lasts for as long as the stimulus is present; after withdrawal of the stimulus, counting is usually resumed. Occasionally, the speech arrest outlasts the actual stimulation.

Walter (in Darley and Millikan 1967: 134) indicated that patients may at times deny having stopped speaking during stimulation. It is as if the currents cause 'a sort of time slip' together with the speech arrest.

Penfield and his team (e.g. Penfield and Rasmussen 1949; Penfield and Roberts 1959: 120–23) reported speech arrests during stimulation in the posterior part of the frontal lobe, the perisylvian area (i.e. the region around the fissure of Sylvius, which separates the parietal from the temporal lobe) and the posterior two-thirds of the second temporal gyrus of the left hemisphere, as well as during stimulation in the lower half of the pre- and post-central gyri (sensorimotor cortex) of the right hemisphere.

Anomia

At times, stimulation does not prevent patients from speaking but makes it difficult for them to name pictures of common objects. The electric pulses interfere with word retrieval, bringing on anomia. Occasionally, the patient involuntarily produces a prolonged or intermittent sound instead of the target word.

Paraphasias and perseverations

It may also happen that the patient misnames the object or the picture shown. The paraphasia may be a perseveration, i.e. the substitution of a previous (correct) answer for the present answer.

Word-finding difficulties, paraphasias and perseverations have been observed during stimulation in the posterior half of the frontal lobe, the perisylvian area and the posterior two thirds of the middle temporal convolution, usually in the left hemisphere. Occasionally, they are noted following stimulation in the anterior part of the temporal lobe or in the parieto-temporo-occipital junction (Ojemann et al. 1989; van Buren et al. 1978)

Iterations, hesitations and slurring

During serial speech (reciting the alphabet or counting aloud), stimulation may cause the patient to repeat a particular item several times in succession. This iteration may last as long as the current is applied. At times, stimulation renders speech delivery laborious or hesitant or causes the patient to speak in a faint voice.

Penfield and Roberts (1959: 122–24) observed iterations, hesitations and slurring during stimulation in the posterior half of the frontal lobe and in the perisylvian area of the left hemisphere, as well as during stimulation in a zone centred around the Rolandic fissure in the right hemisphere (the Rolandic fissure is a vertical fissure separating the frontal from the parietal lobe).

Impaired reading aloud

Electric pulses delivered to the posterior half of the frontal lobe, the perisylvian area and the temporo-parieto-occipital juncture of the left hemisphere may disrupt reading aloud, preventing patients from proceeding with the reading or causing them to produce paralexias. A patient prevented from reading aloud may still be able to speak, as was noted by Morris et al. (1984).

Agraphia

If stimulation is given while patients are writing, the action may be interrupted for as long as the stimulus is applied. During this period, patients may be able to speak, as was noted by Lesser et al. (1984). Speech and writing, then, may be inhibited independently of one another. Agraphia has been observed during stimulation in the posterior part of the frontal and of the temporal lobe on the left.

Impaired short-term verbal memory

Electrostimulation in the temporal and temporo-parietal area of the left hemisphere may impair short-term verbal memory, preventing patients from remembering words that were used a little earlier. Difficulty in remembering words usually varies as a function of the moment at which electrostimulation is given: during input to memory, during storage or during retrieval.

Verbal hallucinations

Interestingly, electrostimulation may also bring on positive symptoms. For instance, stimulation of the temporal cortex may entail verbal hallucinations: patients hear voices or see or hear someone speak, sing or laugh. They may be unable to precisely report what is being said or sung, though.

Involuntary vocalizations

Stimuli applied to the mouth area in the motor cortex of either hemisphere may elicit a sustained vowel sound which continues for as long as stimulation is maintained or until maximum expiration is reached. Then there is a pause for breathing, after which the sound is resumed if stimulation has not ceased. Excitation of the supplementary motor area in the superior part of the mesial aspect of either frontal lobe may result in the production of a prolonged vowel or of a repetitive vowel or syllable. Electrostimulation in the lower part of the motor cortex and in the supplementary motor area, therefore, may bring on negative as well as positive verbal symptoms.

Sustained vocalizations may show more or less rhythmic variations in pitch or volume or else gradual elevation of pitch and/or progressive diminution of volume. Patients are aware of their vocalizations but cannot suppress them. One patient said to the surgeon at the end of a stimulation that had caused loud sound production: 'It felt as though you were pulling the voice out of me' (Penfield 1938).

Involuntary word production

Electric salvoes may also induce involuntary word production. Stimulation of the left amygdala (in the infero-mesial part of the temporal lobe) at times elicits the unintentional utterance of isolated words, which may be repeated several times in succession.

It is worth noticing that electrical stimulation of the convexity (lateral aspect of the hemispheres) has never been reported to induce the production of words.

There is a striking resemblance between the positive and negative symptoms brought on by cortical electrostimulation and the verbal behaviour observed during epileptic seizures (see above, pp. 29–42). Obviously electric pulses delivered during electrostimulation influence language processing in much the same way as epileptic paroxysms do.

Language mapping

The determination of the sites in the cerebral cortex where currents cause negative or positive verbal symptoms is called *(language) mapping* or *functional cortical mapping for language* (see Table 9.1).

However, electric stimulation disrupts or induces linguistic behaviour at different sites in different patients. Indeed, with the possible exception of a small portion of the third frontal convolution just in front of the motor strip, not a single spot has been identified where currents invariably impair verbal performance or elicit sound or word production in all patients. It follows that 'neither the location nor absence of language function at a given cortical site can be reliably predicted by anatomical considerations' (Ojemann et al. 1989). Accordingly, each patient considered for cortectomy or lobectomy in a possibly eloquent area has to be tested individually. Observations made during electrostimulation in one patient are nor unreservedly transferable to another patient.

Moreover, stimulation at a particular point in a particular patient may perturb one verbal activity (say, naming) but leave another activity (say, repetition) intact. In bilinguals, stimulation at a given point may compromise the use of only one language.

Table 9.1: Verbal symptoms brought on by electrostimulation

Sites in the left hemisphere	Verbal symptoms	Sites in the right hemisphere
Posterior half frontal lobe, Perisylvian area Posterior part 2nd temporal gyrus	Speech arrests	Lower half pre- and post-central cortex
Posterior half frontal lobe Perisylvian area Posterior part 2nd temporal gyrus Anterior part temporal lobe (rare) Temporo-parieto-occipital junction	Aphasic disorders	(rare)
Posterior half frontal lobe Perisylvian area	Speech alterations	Area around Rolandic fissure
Posterior half frontal lobe Perisylvian area Temporo-parieto-occipital junction	Reading impairment	
Posterior half frontal lobe Posterior part temporal lobe	Agraphia	
Temporo-parietal area	Verbal memory disturbances	
Temporal lobe	Verbal hallucinations	Temporal lobe
Lower precentral cortex Supplementary motor area	Involuntary vocalizations	Lower precentral cortex Supplementary motor area
Amygdala	Involuntary word production	

There are, then, inter-individual as well as intra-individual differences in response to cortical electrostimulation. Moreover, within a single case, the effect of stimulation is sometimes inconsistent. In a patient described by Ojemann and Whitaker (1978), the same frontal site was stimulated five times during an oral naming task. Three times there resulted a speech arrest, and twice the current failed to disrupt speech production.

Inconsistency in the response of a particular group of neurones to electrostimulation may conceivably be due to the fact that the stimulating probe is usually applied by hand. The manual application is likely to induce slight variations in the pressure exerted by the probe on the cortex and this may influence the neurones' reaction. However, this cannot be the sole cause of variation, since inconsistency has also been observed in patients receiving stimulation via strip electrodes whose pressure on the cortex is invariable.

The sites in a given patient where stimulation causes inhibition or excitation of cerebral language mechanisms are generally discontinuous. In one patient, Ojemann and Whitaker (1978) stimulated three different sites all on the same convolution and within 2 cm of each other. At one site, there were 100 per cent naming errors, while there were no errors at all at the other two sites. In a case reported by Fedio and van Buren (1974), loci were found where naming was correct but where the latency of the responses was unusually long, intermingled with sites where naming was disturbed and sites where it was not. In any subject, then, sites where electrical stimulation interferes with language processing form discrete mosaics whose configurations are highly personal.

Notwithstanding the inter-individual differences, 'eloquent' sites generally lie within the broad fronto-temporo-parietal area where lesions have been found to be located that cause verbal disorders. Occasionally, however, sites of electrical interference are found well outside of the lesion-based perimeter, for instance in the anterior part of the temporal lobe. Indeed, in one study (Bhatnagar and Andy 1983), electrical stimulation in the right hemisphere interfered a number of times with language processing although the Wada test had shown the left hemisphere to be dominant for language.

Cortical excision

Having mapped language in the vicinity of the epileptogenic focus, the neurosurgeon generally removes the sites where there was no reaction to electrostimulation and, as far as possible, spares the sites where electrostimulation interfered with language processing.

This approach is not foolproof, though. Resection of a site where electrostimulation disrupted language does not always result in (durable) verbal impairment. Conversely, there may be (transient) aphasia following excision of portions of the cortex where electrostimulation failed to disturb language processing. Penfield and Roberts have warned (1959: 135) that 'the surgeon must be aware of this possibility'.

The discrepancy sometimes noted between the results of electrostimulation and the consequences of cortical resection may have several causes. Electrical stimuli applied to a small group of neurones may irradiate, through these neurones' projections, to more distant associated neuronal circuits and disturb the performance of these circuits. Such irradiation does not occur when the neurones are removed. On the other hand, surgical ablation is a much more radical procedure than electrostimulation. Therefore, it is not surprising that removal of a stretch of cortex and of part of the underlying whiter matter should at times impair language functioning while electrostimulation of (part of) this stretch did not. Moreover, as a rule, only simple verbal functions such as counting aloud or naming objects on confrontation are assessed during electrical stimulation. Excision may conceivably affect more complex functions which are necessary for the efficient use of language in real communicative situations.

Conclusion

It appears, then, that hemispheric anaesthetization and cortical electrostimulation are useful methods to anticipate the effect of cortical ablation on language. However, they are not completely reliable: excisions of part of the traditional lesion-based language zone within the hemisphere that proved to be dominant for language on the Wada test does not always result in (permanent) language impairment. More importantly, on the other hand, even if there was no aphasia following injection of a barbiturate, cortical ablation may entail (durable) language disorders.

By the same token, response of a given cortical site to electrostimulation does not enable one to predict with complete certainty the effect that resection of this site will have on language. It follows that cortectomy or lobectomy for intractable epilepsy performed in the fronto-temporo-parietal area of the dominant hemisphere always involves the risk of subsequent linguistic deficits. Accordingly, in each case that is being considered for surgery, the pros and cons, the possible gains and likely losses, should be carefully weighed.

CHAPTER 10
Remediation of verbal disorders associated with epilepsy

Epilepsy is usually treated with drugs. It may be necessary to change medication or dosage several times before a favourable effect is obtained. When, despite repeated trials, medication fails to reduce the number and/or the severity of the seizures, neurosurgery is at times resorted to.

In favourable cases, medication or surgery have a beneficial effect not only on epilepsy but also on the verbal disorders that may be associated with it. Indeed, anticonvulsants may occasionally improve verbal performance even in patients who have never presented with seizures and in whom electroencephalography fails to detect paroxysmal discharges, as in the case reported by Guillaume et al. (1957) and discussed above (p. 60).

Unfortunately, there are also cases where language pathology remains (relatively) unaffected by antiepileptic medication and/or surgery. This is particularly so in children with acquired epileptic aphasia (see above, p. 69). More often than not, the little patients continue to suffer from aphasia even if seizures have stopped and EEG recordings have normalized.

Since persistent aphasia seriously compromises the children's scholastic achievements as well as their familial and social integration, verbal therapy is necessary. However, due to the patients' verbal comprehension disorder, giving them therapy is a very difficult task: frequently the little patients fail to understand what the therapist wants them to do. In addition, periods of partial recovery are more than once followed by unexplainable relapses, which is most frustrating for both the patients and their therapists.

If the patient's speech comprehension deficit is part of a more general inability to attach meanings to sounds, an inability known as *auditory agnosia*, therapy often needs to begin at a very basic level. The child must be made to pay attention again to auditory stimuli and try to interpret them.

If despite the child's and the therapist's sustained efforts no substantial progress is achieved, introducing the child to sign language should be seriously considered. This approach, no doubt, will put a tremendous demand on both the patient and their relatives. Learning sign language is by no means an easy task, but it may be the only way out of the dreadful solitude and isolation to which the child is condemned if he/she cannot communicate.

Not only children with acquired but also children with developmental aphasia should be given speech and language therapy, even if the epilepsy, which is often subclinical, is adequately controlled. As a matter of fact, in many of these little patients, subclinical epilepsy is belatedly discovered and treated. In the meantime, the child has failed to develop language normally. Therapy must help him/her catch up as quickly as possible.

Actually, in most cases of verbal disorders associated with epilepsy, speech and language therapy appears indicated, as medication and surgery can at best bring about improvement of verbal performance, but not full recovery.

The only exception, it would seem, is ictal verbal pathology. Obviously, patients cannot be treated during ictal episodes. And since they usually recover all of their linguistic abilities after the seizures, post-ictal therapy appears superfluous. Yet, in children with frequent seizures, linguistic level should be regularly checked, lest the repeated fits in the long run should damage cerebral tissue necessary for efficient language use. Should verbal stagnation or regression be observed, speech and language therapy becomes necessary to avoid further degradation.

Special attention should be given to children who suffer from temporal or frontal lobe epilepsy or have undergone temporal or frontal cortectomy or lobectomy. As was mentioned above (pp. 65, 94), these children may have reduced or underdeveloped metalinguistic skills and/or an impairment of verbal memory. These deficits have to be remedied if they are found to compromise the children's scholastic achievement, particularly as regards the mastery of the mother tongue and the acquisition of foreign languages.

As was shown above (p. 36), diurnal transitory bioelectrical discharges, even if they do not entail observable clinical seizures, may nevertheless cause transient cognitive deficits and may thus interfere with the performance of intellectual tasks, including verbal ones. Schoolchildren with this type of epilepsy are likely to need extra pedagogical support to make for their moments of reduced attention and reduced cognitive performance.

In summary, children suffering from epilepsy and presenting with linguistic deficits should be given verbal therapy. This therapy should continue as long as the deficits are present, even if the epilepsy is eventually adequately controlled. In this connection, it should be remembered that normalization of the EEG recordings cannot be taken as evidence that linguistic problems have cleared up.

Therapy may be desirable even in cases with only nocturnal paroxysms and no clinical manifestations, as such paroxysms may interfere with learning and memorization.

CHAPTER 11

Conclusions

Epilepsy may be associated with a great variety of verbal disorders or deviances. In some cases, epilepsy appears to be the direct cause of the verbal pathology. The abnormal bioelectrical discharges interfere with the processing of speech or language by the brain and thus disrupt the patients' intentional verbal behaviour. At other times, the paroxysmal discharges activate neuronal circuits concerned with language use and elicit involuntary verbal actions of which the patients may or may not be conscious. There is yet a third way in which epilepsy may influence language: repeated seizures may in the long run entail a modification of brain tissue or connectivity and thus hamper the acquisition or efficient use of language.

In some cases, the disturbing discharges are triggered off by the verbal behaviour itself: language induces reflex epilepsy which in turn perturbs language.

At times, the verbal disorders do not result directly from the electrical paroxysms but from the pharmacological or surgical procedure that has been applied in an effort to control the paroxysms.

There are also cases where no causal link can be discovered between language pathology and epilepsy. The two disorders appear to be mere concomitants. They are symptoms of a more general brain disease or damage.

Though very many different verbal shortcomings, disorders, deviances and peculiarities can be observed in people suffering from epilepsy, none of them is typical of the falling sickness: they can all occur in association with other neurological diseases.

Recent observations have shown that epilepsy may reflect negatively on language even if it remains subclinical. Diurnal paroxysms, even though they do not entail clinical seizures, may nevertheless provoke transient cognitive impairments with reduced verbal performance. And continuous spikes and waves during sleep may slow down the development of linguistic skills.

These observations have led some researchers to doubt the appropriateness of the name 'subclinical epilepsy'. This label suggests that epilepsy may

117

take place without interfering with brain functioning. But is this really ever the case? Even those artists who, despite their epilepsy, manage to produce masterpieces present with peculiarities that correlate with their disease.

It appears, then, that epilepsy is a momentous illness that in most cases has a definite influence on the sufferer's verbal behaviour. Indeed, there seem to be few, if any, people with epilepsy whose linguistic competence and/or performance would have been quite the same had they not been plagued by what used to be called in Latin *morbus sonticus* or *morbus maior*, the severe illness, the great malady.

References

Aarts J, Binnie C, Smit A, Wilkins A (1984) Selective cognitive impairment during focal and generalized epileptiform EEG activity. Brain 107: 293-308.

Akelaitis A, Risteen W, Herren Y, van Wegenen W (1942) Studies on the corpus callosum. Archives of Neurology 47: 971-1008.

Alajouanine T (1963) Dostoievski's epilepsy. Brain 86: 209-18.

Alajouanine T, Nehlil J, Gabersek V (1959) A propos d'un cas d'épilepsie déclenchée par la lecture. Revue Neurologique 101: 463-67.

Alajouanine T, Sabouraud O (1960) Les perturbations paroxystiques du langage dans l'épilepsie. L'Encéphale 49: 95-133.

Andermann F (1987) Clinical features of migraine-epilepsy syndromes. In Andermann F, Lugaresi E (eds), Migraine and Epilepsy. Boston: Butterworths. pp 3-30.

Baratz R, Mesulam M (1981) Adult-onset stuttering treated with anticonvulsants. Archives of Neurology 38: 132.

Barbizet J, Degos J, Duizabo P, Chartier B (1974) Syndrome de déconnexion interhémisphérique. Revue Neurologique 130: 127-41.

Bart B (1967) Flaubert. Syracuse: Syracuse University Press.

Baynes E, Kegl J, Brentari D, Kussmaul C, Poizner H (1998) Chronic auditory agnosia following Landau-Kleffner syndrome: a 23 year outcome study. Brain and Language 63: 381-425.

Baynes K, Tramo M, Gazzaniga M (1992) Reading with a limited lexicon in the right hemisphere of a callosotomy patient. Neuropsychologia 30: 187-200.

Bell W, Horner J, Logue P, Radtke R (1990) Neologistic speech automatisms during complex partial seizures. Neurology 40: 49-52.

Bhatnagar S, Andy O (1983) Language in the nondominant right hemisphere. Archives of Neurology 40: 728-31.

Bingley K, Sharp F (1983) Reversible alexia without agraphia due to migraine. Archives of Neurology 40: 114-15.

Blumer D, Benson F (1975) Personality changes with frontal and temporal lobe lesions. In Benson F, Blumer D (eds), Psychiatric Aspects of Neurological Disease. New York: Grune and Stratton. pp 151-69.

Bogen J (1976) Linguistic performance in the short term following cerebral commissurotomy. In Whitaker H (ed.), Studies in Neurolinguistics 2. New York: Academic Press. pp 193-224.

Bogen J, Vogel P (1975) Neurological status in the long term following complete cerebral commissurotomy. In Michel F, Schott B (eds), Les Syndromes de Déconnexion Calleuse chez l'Homme. Lyon: Hôpital Neurologique. pp 227–51.

Bolin B (1953) Left-handedness and stuttering as signs diagnostic of epileptics. Journal of Mental Science 99: 483–88.

Botez M, Wertheim N (1959) Expressive aphasia and amusia. Brain 82: 186–202.

Boudouresque J, Gosset A, Sayag J (1972) Maladie d'Urbach-Wiethe: crises temporales avec phénomènes extatiques et calcification des deux lobes temporaux. Bulletin de l'Académie de Médecine de Paris 156: 416–21.

Brooks J, Jirauch P (1971) Primary reading epilepsy: a misnomer. Archives of Neurology 25: 97–104.

Campbell A, Bogen J, Smith A (1981) Disorganization and reorganization of cognitive and sensorimotor functions in cerebral commissurotomy. Brain 104: 493–511.

Capon A, Huysman E, Moerman C, Toth Q (1973) Manifestations convulsives dans la maladie de Wilson. Archives Suisses de Neurologie, Neurochirurgie et de Psychiatrie 11: 219–25.

Chesni Y (1966) Parole intérieure motrice-kinesthésique et schèmes verbaux intérieurs à caractère auditif: à propos d'une aura hallucinatoire visuelle et auditivo-verbale avec foyer électrographique temporal antérieur droit chez une malade droitière. Revue Neurologique 115: 966–71.

Cirignotta F, Todesco C, Lugaresi E (1980) Temporal lobe epilepsy with ecstatic seizures (so-called Dostoevsky epilepsy). Epilepsia 21: 705–10.

Cohen H, le Normand M (1998) Language development in children with simple-partial left-hemisphere epilepsy. Brain and Language 64: 409–22.

Cole A, Andermann F, Taylor L, Olivier A, Rasmussen T, Robitaille Y, Spire J (1988) The Landau-Kleffner syndrome of acquired aphasia. Neurology 38: 31–38.

Damasio A, Lima A, Damasio H (1975) Nervous function after right hemispherectomy. Neurology 25: 89–93.

Damsté P (1990) Stotteren. Utrecht: Bohn, Scheltema and Holkema.

Darley F, Millikan C (1967) Brain Mechanisms Underlying Speech and Language. New York: Grune and Stratton.

Dennis M, Kohn B (1975) Comprehension of syntax in infantile hemiplegia after cerebral hemidecortication: left hemisphere superiority. Brain and Language 2: 472–82.

Dennis M, Whitaker H (1976) Language acquisition following hemidecortication: linguistic superiority of the left over the right hemisphere. Brain and Language 3: 404–33.

Deonna T, Chevrie C, Hornung E (1987) Childhood epileptic speech disorder: prolonged isolated deficit of prosodic features. Developmental Medicine and Child Neurology 29: 100–105.

du Camp M (1882) Souvenirs Littéraires. Reprinted in 1962. Paris: Hachette.

Dumesnil R (1905) Flaubert, son hérédité, son milieu, sa méthode. Paris, thesis.

Dumesnil R (1947) La maladie et la mort de Flaubert. In Flaubert, l'Homme et l'Oeuvre. Paris: Desclée-De Brouwer.

Ellis A, Young A, Flude B (1987) 'Afferent dysgraphia' in a patient and in normal subjects. Cognitive Neuropsychology 4: 465–86.

Fabbro F (1998) Prospettive d'interpretazione della glossolalia paolina sotto il profilo della neurolinguistica. Revista Biblica 66: 157–78.

Fedio P, van Buren J (1974) Memory deficits following electrical stimulation of the speech cortex in conscious man. Brain and Language 1: 29–42.

Féré C (1905) Le bégaiement épileptique. Revue de Médecine 1: 115–18.

Fleishman J, Segall J, Judge F (1983) Isolated transient alexia: a migrainous accompaniment. Archives of Neurology 40: 115–16.

Foote-Smith E, Bayne L (1991) Joan of Arc. Epilepsia 32: 810–15.

Forster F, Hansotia P, Cleeland C, Ludwig A (1969) A case of voice-induced epilepsy treated with conditioning. Neurology 19: 325–31.

Frank J (1976) Dostoevsky: The Seeds of Revolt. Princeton, NJ: Princeton University Press.

Frank J (1995) Dostoevsky: The Miraculous Years. Princeton, NJ: Princeton University Press.

Freud S (1927) Dostoevsky and parricide. Reproduced in Strachy A, Freud A (eds), The Standard Edition of the Complete Psychological Works of Sigmund Freud. (1961) London: Hogarth.

Garcia-Flores E (1999) Corpus callosotomy for the treatment of Landau-Kleffner syndrome. Epilepsia 40, suppl. 2: 62.

Gastaut H (1978) Fyodor Mikhailovitch Dostoevsky's involuntary contribution to the symptomatology and prognosis of epilepsy. Epilepsia 19: 186–201.

Gastaut H (1979) L'involontaire contribution de Fiodor Mikhaïlovitch Dostoïevski à la symptomatologie et au prognostic de l'épilepsie. L'Evolution Psychiatrique 44: 215–47.

Gastaut H, Gastaut Y (1982) La maladie de Gustave Flaubert. Revue Neurologique 138: 467–92.

Gastaut H, Zifkin B (1984) Ictal visual hallucinations of numerals. Neurology 34: 950–53.

Gates J, Maxwell R, Leppik I, Fiol M, Gumnit R (1985) Electroencephalographic and clinical effects of total corpus callosotomy. In Reeves A (ed.), Epilepsy and the Corpus Callosum. New York: Plenum Press. pp 315–28.

Gazzaniga M, Bogen J, Sperry R (1963) Laterality effects in somesthesis following cerebral commissurotomy in man. Neuropsychologia 1: 209–15.

Gazzaniga M, Bogen J, Sperry R (1967) Dyspraxia following division of the cerebral commissures. Archives of Neurology 16: 606–12.

Gazzaniga M, Sperry R (1967) Language after section of the cerebral commissures. Brain 90: 131–38.

Geschwind N (1984) Dostoievsky's epilepsy. In Blumer D (ed.), Psychiatric Aspects of Epilepsy. Washington, DC: American Psychiatric Press. pp 325–34.

Geschwind N, Sherwin I (1967) Language-induced epilepsy. Archives of Neurology 16: 25–31.

Gordon K, Bawden H, Camfield P, Mann S, Orlik P (1996) Valproic acid treatment of learning disorders and severely epileptiform EEG without clinical seizures. Journal of Child Neurology 11: 41–43.

Griffith H, Davidson M (1966) Long-term changes in intellect and behaviour after hemispherectomy. Journal of Neurology, Neurosurgry, and Psychiatry 29: 571–76.

Guard O, Fournet F, Sautreaux J, Dumas R (1983) Troubles du langage au cours d'une lésion frontale droite chez un droitier: incohérence du discours et paraphasies 'extravagantes'. Revue Neurologique 139: 45–53.

Guillaume J, Mazars G, Mazars Y (1957) Intermédiaire épileptique dans certains types de bégaiement. Revue Neurologique 96: 59–61.

Gur R, Gur R, Sussman N, O'Connor M, Vey M (1984) Hemispheric control of the writing hand. Neurology 34: 904–8.

Hécaen H, Piercy M (1956) Paroxysmal dysphasia and the problem of cerebral dominance. Journal of Neurology, Neurosurgery and Psychiatry 19: 194-201.

Helm N, Butler R, Canter G (1980) Neurogenic acquired stuttering. Journal of Fluency Disorders 5: 269-79.

Herskowitz J, Rosman P, Geschwind N (1984) Seizures induced by singing and recitation: a unique form of reflex epilepsy in childhood. Archives of Neurology 41: 1102-3.

Heuyer G, Feld M (1954) Hémisphérectomie gauche pour atrophie cicatricielle chez un enfant droitier: discussion de l'acquisition postopératoire du langage. Revue Neurologique 90: 52-58.

Hoeppner J, Garrow D, Wilson R, Koch-Weser M (1987) Epilepsy and verbosity. Epilepsia 28: 35-40.

Hurwitz T, Wada J, Kosaka B, Strauss E (1985) Cerebral organisation of affect suggested by temporal lobe seizures. Neurology 35: 1335-37.

Jones R (1966) Observations on stammering after localized cerebral injury. Journal of Neurology, Neurosurgery, and Psychiatry 29: 192-95.

Jones R (1967) Dyspraxic ambiphasia: a neurophysiologic theory of stammering. Transactions of the American Neurological Association 97: 197-201.

Joseph A (1986) A hypergraphic syndrome of automatic writing, affective disorder, and temporal lobe epilepsy in two patients. Journal of Clinical Psychiatry 47: 255-57.

Kapur N (1997) Injured Brains of Medical Minds. Oxford: Oxford University Press.

Kasteleijn-Nols Trenité D, Bakker D, Binnie C, Buerman A, van Raaij M (1988) Psychological effects of subclinical epileptiform EEG discharges, I: Scholastic skills. Epilepsy Research 2: 111-16.

Kutschke G, Brodbeck V, Boor R, Reitter B (1999) Do subclinical epileptic discharges (SED) influence language functions in children with developmental language disorder (DLD)? Epilepsia 40, suppl. 2: 20-21.

Landau W, Kleffner F (1957) Syndrome of acquired aphasia with convulsive disorder in children. Neurology 7: 523-30.

Landsborough D (1987) St. Paul and temporal epilepsy. Journal of Neurology, Neurosurgery, and Psychiatry 50: 659-64.

Laskowitz D, Sperling M, French J, O'Connor M (1995) The syndrome of frontal lobe epilepsy: Characteristics and surgical management. Neurology 45:780-87.

Lebrun Y (1983) Cerebral dominance for language: a neurolinguistic approach. Folia Phoniatrica 35: 13-39.

Lebrun Y (1985) Disturbances of written language and associated abilities following damage to the right hemisphere. Applied Psycholinguistics 6: 231-60.

Lebrun Y (1997a) Adult-onset stuttering. In Lebrun Y (ed.), From the Brain to the Mouth. Dordrecht: Kluwer. pp 105-38.

Lebrun Y (1997b) Subcortical structures and non-volitional verbal behaviour. Journal of Neurolinguistics 10: 313-23.

Lebrun Y (2001) Lalieën en Fasieën. Louvain: Acco.

Lebrun Y, Leleux C (1979) Language functions in hemispherectomized patients. In Lebrun Y, Hoops R (eds), Problems of Aphasia. Lisse: Swets and Zeitlinger. pp 159-73.

Lecours R, Joanette Y (1980) Linguistic and other psychological aspects of paroxysmal aphasia. Brain and Language 10: 1-23.

Lee S, Sutherling W, Persing J, Butler A (1980) Language-induced seizure: a case of cortical origin. Archives of Neurology 37: 433-36.

Leleux C, Lebrun Y (1981) Language development in two cases of left hemispherectomy. In Lebrun Y, Zangwill O (1981) Lateralization of Language in the Child. Lisse: Swets and Zeitlinger. pp 82–88.

Lesser R, Lueders H, Dinner D, Hahn J, Cohen L (1984) The location of speech and writing functions in the frontal language area. Brain 107: 275–91.

McFie J (1961) The effect of hemispherectomy on intellectual functioning in cases of infantile hemiplegia. Journal of Neurology, Neurosurgery, and Psychiatry 24: 240–49.

Madison D, Baeher E, Bazell M, Hartmann K, Mahurkar S, Dunea G (1977) Communicative and cognitive deterioration in dialysis dementia: two case studies. Journal of Speech and Hearing Disorders 42: 238–346.

Manders E, Bastijns P (1988) Sudden recovery from stuttering after an epileptic attack: a case report. Journal of Fluency Disorders 13: 421–25.

Marescaux C, Hirsch E, Finck S, Maquet P, Schlumberger E, Sellal F, Metz-Lutz M, Alembik Y, Salmon E, Franck G, Kurtz D (1990) Landau-Kleffner syndrome: a pharmacological study of five cases. Epilepsia 31: 768–77.

Marino R, Ragazzo P (1985) Selective criteria and results of selective partial callosotomy. In Reeves A (ed.), Epilepsy and the Corpus Callosum. New York: Plenum Press. pp 281–301.

Marsh G (1978) Neuropsychological syndrome in a patient with episodic howling and violent motor behaviour. Journal of Neurology, Neurosurgery, and Psychiatry 41: 366–69.

Martin R, Loring D, Meador K, Lee G (1990) The effects of lateralized temporal lobe dysfunction on formal and semantic word fluency. Neuropsychologia 29: 823–29.

Mayeux R, Brandt J, Rosen J, Benson F (1980) Interictal memory and language impairment in temporal lobe epilepsy. Neurology 30: 120–26.

Mazars G, Hécaen H, Tzavaras A, Merienne L (1970) Contribution à la chirurgie de certains bégaiements et à la compréhension de leur physiopathologie. Revue Neurologique 122: 213–20.

McClean M, McLean A (1985) Case report of stuttering acquired in association with phenytoin use for post head injury seizures. Journal of Fluency Disorders 10: 241–56.

Meyer F, Marsh R, Laws E, Sharbrough F (1986) Temporal lobectomy in children with epilepsy. Journal of Neurosurgery 64: 371–76.

Mikati M, Saab R (2000) Successful use of intravenous immunoglobin as initial monotherapy in Landau-Kleffner syndrome. Epilepsia 41: 880–86.

Milner B, Branch C, Rasmussen T (1964) Observations on cerebral dominance. In de Reuck A, O'Connor M (eds), Disorders of Language. London: Churchill. pp 200–14.

Miller A (1985) Cessation of stuttering with progressive multiple sclerosis. Neurology 35: 1341–43.

Morrell F, Whisler W, Smith M, Hoeppner T, Toledo-Morrell L, Pierre-Louis S, Kanner A, Buelow J, Ristanovic R, Bergen D, Hasegawa H (1995) Landau-Kleffner syndrome: treatment with subpial intracortical transection. Brain 118: 1529–46.

Morris H, Luders H, Lesser R, Dinner D, Hahn J (1984) Transient neuropsychological abnormalities (including Gerstmann's syndrome) during cortical stimulation. Neurology 34: 877–83.

Murai T, Hanakawa T, Sengoku A, Ban T, Yoneda Y, Fujita H, Fugita N (1998) Temporal lobe epilepsy in a genius of natural history. Neurology 50: 1373–76.

Nagafuchi M, Inuma K, Yamamoto K, Kitamara T (1993) Diazepam therapy of verbal auditory agnosia. Brain and Language 45: 180–88.

Nass R, Gross A, Wisoff J, Devinsky O (1999) Outcome of multiple pial transection for autistic epileptiform regression. Pediatric Neurology 21: 464–70.

Novelly R, Augustine E, Mattson R, Glaser G, Williamson P, Spencer D, Spencer S (1984) Selective memory improvement and impairment in temporal lobectomy for epilepsy. Annals of Neurology 15: 64–67.

Novelly R, Lifrak M (1985) Forebrain commissurotomy reinstates effects of preexisting hemispheric lesions. In Reeves A (ed.), Epilepsy and the Corpus Callosum. New York: Plenum Press. pp 467–500.

Ogden J (1996) Phonological dyslexia and phonological dysgraphia following left and right hemispherectomy. Neuropsychologia 34: 905–18.

Ojemann G, Dodrill C (1985) Verbal memory deficits after left temporal lobectomy for epilepsy. Journal of Neurosurgery 62: 101–7.

Ojemann G, Ojemann J, Lettich E, Berger M (1989) Cortical language localization in left dominant hemisphere. Journal of Neurosurgery 71: 316–26.

Ojemann G, Whitaker H (1978) The bilingual brain. Archives of Neurology 35: 409–12.

Orton S (1927) Studies in stuttering. Archives of Neurology and Psychiatry 18: 671–72.

Orton S (1928) A physiological theory of reading disability and stuttering in children. New England Journal of Medicine 9: 97–113.

Palmini A, Gloor P, Jones-Gotman M (1992) Pure amnestic seizures in temporal lobe epilepsy. Brain 115: 749–69.

Penfield W (1938) The cerebral cortex in man, I: the cerebral cortex and consciousness. Archives of Neurology and Psychiatry 40: 417–42.

Penfield W, Rasmussen T (1949) Vocalization and arrest of speech. Archives of Neurology and Psychiatry 61: 21–27.

Penfield W, Roberts L (1959) Speech and Brain Mechanisms. Princeton, NJ: Princeton University Press.

Penfield W, Welch K (1951) The supplementary motor area of the cerebral cortex. Archives of Neurology and Psychiatry 66: 289–317.

Picard A, Cheliout Heraut F, Brouskraoui M, Lemoine M, Lacert P, Delattre J (1998) Sleep EEG and developmental dysphasia. Developmental Medicine and Child Neurology 40: 595–99.

Platz T (1996) Tactile agnosia: casuistic evidence and theoretical remarks on modality-specific meaning, representation and sensorimotor integration. Brain 119: 1565–74.

Ramani V (1991) Audiogenic epilepsy induced by a specific television performer. New England Journal of Medicine 325: 134–35.

Risse G, Gates J, Lund G, Maxwell R, Rubens A (1989) Interhemispheric transfer in patients with incomplete section of the corpus callosum. Archives of Neurology 46: 437–43.

Roberts D (1985) Corpus callosotomy. In Reeves A (ed.), Epilepsy and the Corpus Callosum. New York: Plenum Press. pp 259–67.

Roberts J, Robertson M, Trimble M (1982) The lateralizing significance of hypergraphia in temporal lobe epilepsy. Journal of Neurology, Neurosurgery, and Psychiatry 45: 131–38.

Ronen G, Richards J, Cunningham C, Secord M, Rosembloom D (2000) Can sodium valproate improve learning in children with epileptiform bursts but without clinical seizures? Developmental Medicine and Child Neurology 42: 751–55.

Rosenbek J, McNeil M, Prescott T, Alfrey A (1975) Speech and language findings in a chronic hemodialysis patient: a case report. Journal of Speech and Hearing Disorders 40: 245–52.

Ross M, Reeves A, Roberts D (1984) Postcommissurotomy mutism. Annals of Neurology 16: 114.

Sartre J (1971) L'Idiot de la Famille. Paris: Gallimard.

Sass K, Novelly R, Spencer D, Spencer S (1990) Postcallosotomy language impairments in patients with crossed cerebral dominance. Journal of Neurosurgery 72: 85-90.

Satz P, Bullard-Bates C (1981) Acquired aphasia in children. In Taylor Sarno M (ed.), Acquired Aphasia. New York: Academic Press. pp 399-426.

Schmidt R, Wilder J (1968) Epilepsy. Philadelphia: Davis.

Schwartz M (1994) Ictal language shift in a polyglot. Journal of Neurology, Neurosurgery, and Psychiatry 57: 121.

Serafetinides E, Falconer M (1963) Speech disturbances in temporal lobe seizures: a study of 100 epileptic patients submitted to anterior temporal lobectomy. Brain 86: 333-46.

Siebelink B, Bakker D, Binnie C, Kasteleijn-Nolst Trenité D (1988) Psychological effects of subclinical epileptiform EEG discharges in children, II: general intelligence tests. Epilepsy Research 2: 117-21.

Sirigu A, Duhamel J, Poncet M (1991) The role of sensorimotor experience in object recognition. Brain 114: 2555-73.

Souques A. (1928) Note sur les troubles de l'écriture pendant les absences épileptiques et sur l'intérêt psychologique et médico-légal de ces troubles. Revue Neurologique 1: 353-60.

Sperry R, Gazzaniga M, Bogen J (1969) Interhemispheric relationships: the neocortical commissures; syndromes of hemispheric disconnection. In Vinken P, Bruyn G (eds), Handbook of Clinical Neurology. Amsterdam: North-Holland Publishing Company. pp 273-90.

Stevens H (1957) Reading epilepsy. New England Journal of Medicine 257: 165-70.

Subirana A (1958) The prognosis of aphasia in relation to cerebral dominance and handedness. Brain 81: 415-25.

Sutherling W, Hershman L, Miller J, Lee S (1980) Seizures induced by playing music. Neurology 30: 1001-4.

Taylor D, Marsh S (1980) Hughlings Jackson's Dr. Z: the paradigm of temporal lobe epilepsy revealed. Journal of Neurology, Neurosurgery, and Psychiatry 43: 758-67.

Terzano M, Parrino L, Manzoni G, Mancia D (1983) Seizures triggered by blinking when beginning to speak. Archives of Neurology 40: 103-6.

Travis L (1978) The cerebral dominance theory of stuttering: 1931-1978. Journal of Speech and Hearing Disorders 43: 278-81.

Tsuru T, Mori M, Mizuguchi M, Momoi M (2000) Effects of high-dose intravenous corticosteroid therapy in Landau-Kleffner syndrome. Pediatric Neurology 22: 145-47.

Tsuzuki H, Kasuga I (1978) Paroxysmal discharges triggered by hearing spoken language. Epilepsia 19: 147-54.

Tuchman R (1994) Epilepsy, language, and behaviour: clinical models in childhood. Journal of Child Neurology 9: 95-102.

van Bogaert L (1934) Ocular paroxysms and palilalia. Journal of Nervous and Mental Disease 80: 48-61.

van Buren J, Fedio P, Frederick G (1978) Mechanism and localization of speech in the parietotemporal cortex. Neurosurgery 2: 233-39.

van Dongen H, van Harskamp F, van Loonen M (1977) Verworven afasie bij kinderen. Nederlands Tijdschrift voor Geneeskunde 121: 813-16.

van Riper C (1971) The Nature of Stuttering. Englewood Cliffs, NJ: Prentice-Hall.

Vharga-Khadem F, Carr L, Isaacs E, Brett E, Adams C, Mishkin M (1997) Onset of speech after left hemispherectomy in a nine-year-old boy. Brain 120: 159–82.

Waxman S, Geschwind N (1975) The inter-ictal behavior of temporal lobe epilepsy. Archives of General Psychiatry 32: 1580–1506.

West R (1958) An agnostic's speculations about stuttering. In Eisenson J (ed.), Stuttering: A Symposium. New York: Harper and Row. pp 167–222.

Wernicke C (1874) Der Aphasische Symptomencomplex. Breslau: Cohn and Weigert.

Wilson M, McNaughton B (1994) Reactivation of hippocampal ensemble memories during sleep. Science 265: 676–79.

Wohlfart G, Ingvar D, Hellberg A (1961) Compulsory shouting (Benedek's 'klazomania') associated with oculogyric spasms in chronic epidemic encephalitis. Acta Psychiatrica et Neurologica Scandinavica 36: 369–77.

Zaidel E (1990) Language functions in the two hemispheres following complete cerebral commissurotomy and hemispherectomy. In Boller F, Grafman J (eds), Handbook of Neuropsychology 4. Amsterdam: Elsevier. pp 115–49.

Zaidel E, Oxbury S, Oxbury J (1994) Effects of surgery in unilateral medial temporal lobe regions on verbal explicit and implicit memory. Neuropsychiatry, Neuropsychology, and Behavioral Neurology 7: 104–8.

Index